GOOD | BAD
FAT | FAT

linoleic - omega 6
alpha - linoleic omega 3

GOOD | BAD
FAT | FAT

LOUISE LAMBERT-LAGACÉ
and
MICHELLE LAFLAMME

First published in 1995 by
Stoddart Publishing Co. Limited
34 Lesmill Road
Toronto, Canada
M3B 2T6
(416) 445-3333

Stoddart Books are available for bulk purchase for sales promotions, premiums, fundraising, and seminars. For details, contact the Special Sales Department at the above address.

Some of the material in this book first appeared by the same authors in French under the title *Bons Gras, Mauvais Gras* in 1993 and was translated by Brian Sparkes, Ph.D.

Canadian Cataloguing in Publication Data

Lambert-Lagacé, Louise, 1941–
Good fat, bad fat

Translation of: Bons gras, mauvais gras.
Includes index.
ISBN 0-7737-5713-9

I. Food – Fat content. 2. Cholesterol. 3. Oils and fats, Edible. I. Laflamme, Michelle. II. Title

TX560.F3L3513 1995   613.2'8   C95-930068-6

Cover Photo: Pierre Tison
Cover Design: General Theory
Computer Graphics: Tannice Goddard

Printed and bound in Canada

Stoddart Publishing gratefully acknowledges the support of the Canada Council, Ontario Ministry of Culture, Tourism, and Recreation, Ontario Arts Council, and Ontario Publishing Centre in the development of writing and publishing in Canada.

CONTENTS

ACKNOWLEDGMENTS

This book took five years to prepare and involved the generous assistance of many people. Since 1989, patients at our nutrition clinic gave us the feedback we needed to establish the basic questions and concerns. Josée Thibodeau, a dietitian and our research assistant since 1992, worked intensively on all segments of the manuscript. Her excellent ideas and thoughtful remarks made quite a difference.

Professors Victor Gavino and Guylaine Ferland of the Department of Nutrition at the University of Montreal, Stan Kubow of McGill University, and Mohsen Meydani of Tufts University in Boston were invaluable collaborators in our series of analyses of cold-pressed oil. Bernard Stier of Maison Orphée of Québec and Jim Dick of Canamara Foods of Saskatchewan also provided unique help in this exciting venture.

Monik St-Pierre, Isabelle Gohier, and André Lamothe, students in dietetics, collected information on food labels in many cities and spent hours in university libraries completing the bibliographic research. Isabelle Vachon kindly illustrated the different fatty acids.

Louise Desaulniers, our associate, reviewed and skillfully critiqued the first edition of the manuscript.

We solicited major scientists around the country to critique this edition. Their willingness to go through every page of the manuscript was greatly appreciated, and their reactions were most helpful. Thank you Dr. Kenneth K. Carroll of the University of Western Ontario, Dr. Bruce McDonald at the University of Manitoba, and Dr. Stan Kubow and Dr. Harriett Kuhnlein of McGill University for your exceptional support.

Anne Lindsay, the renowned cook and a wonderful friend, provided a very meaningful quote for the back cover. What a treat!

Our life companions, Guy Bourgeault and Maurice Lagacé,

worked on the charts, revised the text and graphics, and were most patient with the authors.

Nelson Doucet at Stoddart believed in the book and bought it. Brian Sparkes translated the manuscript patiently and faithfully. Elsha Leventis edited the manuscript with tender loving care, as always.

We are most grateful to all our collaborators and supporters.

INTRODUCTION

Bad fat is slipping onto our plates and it's high time we noticed. Our health depends on it.

The fear of cholesterol has taken on decidedly exaggerated proportions, yet recent research is telling us that margarine and other hydrogenated fats — fats we thought were safe — are also hazardous to our health. Meanwhile fat-free salad dressings, cholesterol-free croissants, and light cheeses proliferate in a clamor of contradictory messages.

We are bombarded by new theories. Confusion reigns.

Should we go back to butter before we have the last word on margarine? Should we buy cholesterol-free oils or cold-pressed oils? Should we indulge in foods labeled "fat free" and splurge on low-fat ice cream? Should we follow the French, who seem to tolerate high intakes of fat better than we do, and wash down our meals with red wine?

This book provides answers and clarifications but, more importantly, introduces a new perspective based on the latest scientific information.

While most health authorities recommend reducing the *quantities* of fat in our diet, we emphasize choosing the right *quality* of fat. While some nutritionists hesitate to qualify individual foods as good or bad for you, we feel doing so is only common sense. When a food has high nutritional value, is useful to most body cells, and presents no potential problem, we call it a *good* food. When a food has poor nutritional value and causes more harm than good, we call it a *bad* food.

Good fats are fats that are essential to cellular growth, development, and maintenance; they provide definite health benefits and don't trigger any harmful reactions in our bodies. They are best when they have undergone minimum transformation during processing.

Bad fats are fats that have been processed to the extent that they have lost their original composition and behavior. They disturb the body's natural way of processing fats. They have also been shown to cause trouble in the arteries as well as in the immune system.

Some fats are neither good nor bad according to our definitions; they are naturally present in certain foods and may cause problems when eaten in excess. Our golden rule (chapter 5) will help you sort them out.

We admit to having changed our views over the years.

Louise: "In one of my previous books, published in 1977, I sharply criticized the overconsumption of meat and fat, but I encouraged the use of corn oil and margarine. At the time, corn oil (a polyunsaturated oil) was used in medical research and was advocated to reduce cholesterol. The ill effects of the hydrogenation of oils were still widely unrecognized in the scientific world. The scientific data have made a major shift during the eighties. In 1988, to be consistent with these new findings and with my new convictions, I asked my publisher not to reprint that book. Since that time I have been working with my associate Michelle Laflamme to shape the present work."

Michelle: "I always dreamed of knowing everything about everything. The subject proposed by Louise came at the right time. I wanted to know more about cardiovascular disease, which took both my father and mother. I wanted to learn more about the link between this health problem and the food we eat. Cholesterol being under fire, I wanted to find out precisely why. Research on cholesterol led me to study other dietary fats; and research on other dietary fats led me to their connection with cancer, autoimmune diseases, and weight problems. I learned quite a lot — and some of it was quite surprising — but have to admit I have not found definite answers to all my questions."

After five years of reviewing the scientific literature, coordinating a series of laboratory analyses on cold-pressed oils, and checking many foods on the market, we wish to share with you our global evaluation.

Although we help you understand the difference between blood cholesterol and food cholesterol, our review goes way beyond the traditional fat and heart connection. We look at cancer, weight problems, and lack of immunity as they relate to fat.

We present friendly definitions of all the different fats so that you can feel at ease with the scientific jargon concerning saturated, monounsaturated, polyunsaturated, and hydrogenated fats.

We provide a critical analysis of the new food labels and health claims to help you become immune to all sorts of misleading messages.

We introduce a new golden rule based on a wide range of fresh or hardly processed foods that can supply your daily dose of good fat.

We offer practical advice on how to choose and serve good fats, how to cook fats at home, and what to eat in restaurants.

We've tried our best to make things simple, but we realize that the whole issue of fats is extremely complex and in constant evolution. Although we don't have the final word, we believe we're on the right track. Our approach is a healthful, common-sense approach; it definitely advocates less processed fats and sets quality as the first priority.

You don't have to have "high blood cholesterol" to be interested in good fats and bad fats. It's a matter of health.

I

For Better...

Nutrition experts criticize, and rightly so, our excessive consumption of fat, but they rarely emphasize the vital role certain fats play. We need only a minute amount of fat, but we cannot function properly without it.

The role of fats in general

Dietary fats not only give flavor to foods, they also supply calories, in fact, more calories than any other nutrient. A tablespoon (15 ml) of oil supplies 124 calories; a tablespoon of sugar only 50. Each time we swallow a gram of fat we take in 9 calories; each time we eat the same amount of sugar we get 4. While 15 milliliters (1 tbsp) of butter contains 11 grams of fat and has 100 calories, whole-wheat bread contains little fat, and one slice supplies 80 calories. Dietary fats, both visible and hidden, do provide many calories, but they must not be totally avoided — it's a matter of health.

Dietary fats also serve as a means of transportation for vitamins A, D, E, and K. Eating a small amount of visible fat or foods that contain fat is absolutely essential to allow the body to use these vitamins efficiently. This applies whether these four vitamins are taken in the form of supplements or in natural foods.

Among all the different fats in our food supply, two have been labeled essential because they cannot be manufactured by the human body itself; they must be supplied by the foods we eat. They are linoleic acid and alpha-linolenic acid. For many years they were called vitamin F and are still sometimes identified this way in Europe.

The role of essential fatty acids

Nutrition experts began the slow process of determining the role of these two essential fatty acids about the end of the twenties. Having fed different diets containing no essential fatty acids to laboratory animals, researchers observed the appearance of several symptoms, such as growth retardation, eczema, reduction in fertility, and decreased visual acuity.

At the beginning of the sixties, other researchers found that a baby fed only intravenously showed serious skin problems after a few weeks. Laboratory tests having shown almost no linoleic acid in the child's serum, the researchers looked more closely at the infant's tube-fed formula and noticed it was virtually fat-free and therefore contained no essential fatty acids.

In those days experts believed that linoleic acid was the only essential fatty acid humans needed. They knew that alpha-linolenic acid was necessary in several animal species for the development of the brain and the retina of the eye and that it ensured the survival of salmon, trout, and certain insects. Nevertheless they were unaware of its essential role in humans.

Then, in the early eighties, researchers observed the symptoms of deficiency in a six-year-old girl who was fed intravenously for five months. During these months, the little girl suffered from extreme weakness, numbness, inability to walk, and cloudy vision. When the American scientist Ralph Holman and his collaborators at the Hormel Institute in Minnesota analyzed all the ingredients and nutrients in the liquid formula, they realized that the only possible missing nutrient was alpha-linolenic acid. Once they added this second essential fatty acid to the formula, the girl's symptoms disappeared very quickly.

We now know that these two essential fatty acids help maintain the integrity of all body cells, whether nerve cells, liver cells, or skin cells. They make sure that each cell is well wrapped in a thin fluid fat membrane that protects the cell's contents and ensures good nutrient exchanges among all the different cells.

From conception on, the fetus needs essential fatty acids. During pregnancy, the fats fed to the fetus through the red blood cells of the placenta are directly influenced by the mother's diet. A diet deficient in essential fatty acids affects the development of the placenta, which in turn retards the growth of the fetus, as well as the development of the brain and the nervous system. Studies have shown that mothers who gave birth to low-birth-weight babies consumed fewer essential fatty acids (5.5 grams compared with 12 grams per day) than mothers who gave birth to babies weighing more than 2.5 kilograms (5.5 pounds) at birth.

Once the baby is born, an adequate amount of essential fatty acids is also needed, since the brain develops exceedingly rapidly during the first twelve months of life, and since 60 percent of the brain's solid matter is composed of essential fatty acids. Breast milk contains up to seven times more essential fatty acids than cow's milk. Breast milk also contains adequate amounts of a derivative of alpha-linolenic acid called DHA, which plays a crucial role in the development of the brain and the retina of the eye. Since premature and very low-birth-weight babies cannot manufacture this derivative (normal-weight babies, children, and adults can) and since fatty acids can make a long-term difference in the IQ and visual acuity of premature babies, infant-formula companies are actually going back to the drawing board once more to improve the fat content of their formulas.

A study involving twenty-two children with cystic fibrosis at St. Justine Hospital in Montreal showed that essential fatty acids were indispensable for ensuring the adequate transportation of cholesterol and other fats in the blood.

Linoleic acid is the parent substance of the omega-6 family, while alpha-linolenic acid is the parent substance of the omega-3 family. All through the life cycle, these two parent substances produce two series of derivatives that become chemical messengers called prostaglandins. Prostaglandins act rapidly at very precise sites in the body and allow the proper functioning of the circulatory, immune, anti-inflammatory, and epithelial systems, among others. In other words, essential fatty acids help manage our blood, our antibodies, our hormones, and our skin. To accomplish their vital activities, the two essential fatty acids need to be present in the food we eat, but they also need to be transported and transformed properly. Yet to do so, they must compete with other fats, which also need to be transported and transformed. If, for example, we eat tons of cheese, fried foods, crackers, and margarine and very few whole grains, leafy green vegetables, nuts, and fish, the fats in the first group of foods will compete with and easily win over the essential fatty acids in the second. Without a fair balance of linoleic acid and alpha-linolenic acid in our diet, the production of their derivatives and of the prostaglandins can be compromised, provoking such problems as abnormal sugar metabolism, atherosclerosis, hypertension, and other debilitating diseases. "Optimal health depends on an optimal ratio of the two essential fatty acids," underlined Edward Siguel and Robert Lerman of the Boston University Medical Center Hospital in one of their recent research publications.

Those who might be lacking essential fatty acids

Growing children need essential fatty acids for the growth and development of all tissues. Even plumpness is no grounds for cutting fat completely from their diets. Children's growth and puberty can be adversely affected if they are submitted to severe fat restrictions.

Women who follow very strict weight-reducing diets or eat very little food can suffer a lack of essential fatty acids. If, for example, they avoid all whole-grain cereal products, nuts and seeds, and legumes, or cut out all visible fat — even the smallest drop of oil in a salad — they can develop dry skin, experience difficult and irregular periods, have trouble becoming pregnant, and go through an exhausting menopause. Symptoms can get even worse if a person has the eating disorder anorexia nervosa.

Patients with chronic malabsorption problems, as in the case of severe gastrointestinal disease (celiac or Crohn's disease), have been shown to be truly deficient in essential fatty acids, but even less severe conditions such as gastric ulcers can also be linked to a lack of essential fatty acids. In 1986, D. Hollander of Oxford University and A. Tarnawski of the University of California noted that there was a parallel between an increased consumption of linoleic acid (one of the two essential fatty acids) and the decreased incidence and gravity of peptic ulcers. They then suggested that additional linoleic acid could protect gastric tissues by increasing the production of protective prostaglandins. Since then, many researchers have attempted to verify the hypothesis. At the University of Edinburgh, Dr. H. Grant and his associates recruited thirty-five men suffering from ulcers and thirty-five healthy men and analyzed the fat tissue just under their skin to measure the content of linoleic acid. While the composition of fat tissue in individuals quite faithfully reflects the amount of fat in their diets, they noted that the percentage of linoleic acid was lower among the men with ulcers. This study showed that men afflicted with ulcers retained less linoleic acid than healthy men. The full impact of this study is yet to be determined.

Textbooks on nutrition and medicine consider human essential fatty-acid deficiency an extremely rare disorder that is usually associated with tube-fed patients not receiving fat supplements. This longstanding belief is currently being challenged.

Cardiac patients are another vulnerable group. A team of British scientists recently analyzed the tissue taken at autopsy from eighty-four male victims of sudden cardiac death and compared their results with the same analyses done on 230 healthy individuals living in the South West Hampshire Health District. Lower levels of linoleic acid were found in the tissues of the victims than in those of the healthy volunteers. The authors believe that clinical and experimental evidence is now sufficient to show that a relative deficiency of essential fatty acid is related to coronary heart disease.

Edward Siguel and Robert Lerman conducted a different study in Boston among confirmed cardiac patients and compared specific blood values with those of healthy volunteers. Their study reveals that cardiac patients have an essential fatty-acid insufficiency that can exacerbate their cardiovascular disease by forcing the cells to incorporate more cholesterol, which can harden the walls of the blood vessels. This mild deficiency is not necessarily caused by a lack of fat in the diet but by a diet loaded with animal fat and vegetable shortenings, which interfere with the cells' access to essential fatty acids. "A large segment of the U.S. population eats mainly processed foods which are deficient in essential fatty acids," Dr. Siguel said in an interview published in the *Nutrition Post.*

The elderly can also be at risk of a deficiency in essential fatty acids. A study carried out in Dijon revealed low blood levels of essential fatty acids among an elderly population eating small amounts of food. Inadequate food intake limits the availability of essential fatty acids, and the normal aging process causes a decrease in the body's ability to absorb these fatty acids, two conditions that affect the production of the derivatives and their prostaglandins, which in turn increase the risk of circulatory problems and arthritic pain.

More and more evidence is piling in that highly processed fats, along with the fats in meats and cheeses, are seriously competing with the two essential fatty acids, preventing them from following their natural game plan, thus creating a new form of deficiency.

The renowned U.K. scientist Hugh Sinclair, in a 1956 letter published in *Lancet*, one of the most respected scientific journals, emphasized that *the majority of modern diseases could be due to a deficiency in essential fatty acids or to a problem of their transformation during processing.* Fats have been under scrutiny ever since, and many researchers are now confirming some of Sinclair's worries, but "truth is the daughter of time and not of authority."

The omega-3 fatty acids

As mentioned above, alpha-linolenic acid is the parent substance for a large family of fatty acids called the omega-3 fatty acids. These fatty acids have become quite famous in recent years; they are found mainly in seafood, but are also present in linseed oil, walnuts, canola oil, soybeans, soya oil, and dark green leafy vegetables. Specialists are now using these fatty acids to improve the treatment of certain illnesses.

At the University of Alberta, researchers in gastrointestinal diseases (Crohn's disease and ulcerative colitis) found that omega-3 fatty acids from fish oils decreased intestinal inflammation in laboratory animals.

At Mount Sinai Medical Center in New York, doctors used fish oil rich in omega-3 fatty acids to treat ten patients with colitis. After a period of eight weeks, they found a definite improvement in seven patients and no change among the other three. Research is still going on in this area.

At University Hospital in Montreal, a fish-oil supplement rich in omega-3 fatty acids, given for three months to a small group of patients with genetically high blood cholesterol, showed that omega-3 fatty acids prevented a rapid increase in blood cholesterol levels and could delay the risk of premature atherosclerosis in such a vulnerable group.

Elsewhere, people who eat fish frequently seem to have less chronic inflammatory diseases than North Americans. In Denmark, researchers wanting to verify this observation measured the impact of a fish-oil supplement given for twelve weeks to people suffering from rheumatoid arthritis and compared the results with a control group given a placebo containing no fish oil. They found there was a net improvement in those patients taking the fish oil and concluded that omega-3 fatty acids could be a useful complement to traditional therapies for this kind of arthritis.

At the Royal Adelaide Hospital in Australia, healthy volunteers were fed a diet rich in linseed oil to see if a vegetable oil rich in omega-3 fatty acid could be as efficient as a fish-oil supplement. The results were conclusive, and the authors of this study advised that the regular consumption of linseed oil could be a primary health measure for chronic conditions such as coronary heart disease, or in inflammatory diseases such as rheumatoid arthritis and colitis.

Another study published in 1991 dealt with the influence of alpha-linolenic acid on the immune systems of ten American subjects. The study used linseed oil as an excellent source of alpha-linolenic acid, and the results prompted the researchers to believe that this oil could be useful in the treatment of autoimmune or chronic inflammatory diseases such as arthritis, lupus, and allergies.

In 1992, Corrine Benquet of the University of Quebec in Montreal, compared the impact of five different fats on the immune system of mice undergoing intense exercise. Normally such stress in Olympic athletes affects the production of antibodies and forces some athletes to withdraw from competition to prevent more serious complications. Linseed oil rich in alpha-linolenic acid was the only fat that maintained the production of antibodies in the study on mice.

Scientists from the National Health Foundation looked at omega-3 fatty acids and their impact on human breast-cancer growth using a mouse model system. After comparing a diet rich in corn oil (low in omega-3 fatty acids) with one rich in fish oil (high in omega-3 fatty acids), they concluded that a diet rich in omega-3 fatty acids could suppress human breast-cell growth and metastases in mice. The authors, David Rose and Jeanne Connolly, suggest that dietary intervention trials to reduce the risk of recurrence in postsurgical breast-cancer patients should take into account not only the quantities of fat consumed but also the *quality* of the fatty acids used.

In France, a team of scientists made the headlines in June 1994 with their successful clinical trial aimed at preventing a second heart attack among cardiac patients during the first two years after their first attack. Their diet included a higher content of alpha-linolenic acid to imitate the Mediterranean diet, and the results showed a dramatic reduction in mortality when compared with other trials. Alpha-linolenic acid seems to have made the difference.

Another study carried out among 8,960 current or former smokers measured the impact of omega-3 fatty acids on chronic respiratory-system diseases and concluded that an adequate dietary intake of omega-3 fatty acids may protect against chronic bronchitis and emphysema in such a population.

You may have noticed that all these success stories are based on the right *quality* of fatty acids, not on the reduction of the total quantity of fat.

The essential fatty acids in our basic foods

Table 1 contains a list of common foods and their content of fats and essential fatty acids. To familiarize yourself with the fat content of the major food groups, you should study this list.

Table 1
Essential fatty acid content of some foods

FOOD	PORTION	FAT (g)	ESSENTIAL FATTY ACIDS linoleic (g)	alpha-linolenic (g)
CEREAL PRODUCTS				
amaranth	125 ml/1/2 c	6.4	2.8	0.06
oats	125 ml/1/2 c	5.4	1.9	0.09
corn	125 ml/1/2 c	3.9	1.7	0.05
millet	125 ml/1/2 c	1.2	0.6	0.03
barley	125 ml/1/2 c	2.1	0.9	0.10
cooked brown rice	250 ml/1 c	1.8	0.6	0.03
cooked wild rice	250 ml/1 c	0.6	0.2	0.16
wheat germ	60 ml/4 tbsp	2.8	1.5	0.21
whole-wheat flour	125 ml/1/2 c	1.1	0.4	0.02
cooked whole-wheat pasta	250 ml/1 c	0.8	0.3	0.02
granola breakfast cereal	60 ml/4 tbsp	7.9	3.9	0.2
FRUITS AND VEGETABLES				
avocado	half	15	1.9	0.1
other fruits	250 ml/1 c	0.5	0.1	0.05
vegetables	250 ml/1 c	0.3	0.1	0.05

FOOD	PORTION	FAT (g)	ESSENTIAL FATTY ACIDS	
			linoleic (g)	alpha-linolenic (g)
OILS				
canola	15 ml/1 tbsp	13.5	3.0	1.5
safflower	15 ml/1 tbsp	13.5	10.1	0.1
wheat germ	15 ml/1 tbsp	13.5	7.5	0.9
linseed	15 ml/1 tbsp	13.5	1.7	7.3
corn	15 ml/1 tbsp	13.5	7.9	0.1
walnut	15 ml/1 tbsp	13.5	7.2	1.4
olive	15 ml/1 tbsp	13.5	1.1	0.1
grape seed	15 ml/1 tbsp	13.5	9.5	traces
soya	15 ml/1 tbsp	13.5	6.9	0.9
sunflower	15 ml/1 tbsp	13.5	8.9	0.9
MEAT AND OTHER PROTEIN SOURCES				
egg	1 medium	6	0.6	0.02
veal	100 g/3 oz	11	0.2	0.14
halibut	100 g/3 oz	2.8	0.04	0.10
crab	100 g/3 oz	2	0.1	0.17
cooked soy beans	250 ml/1 c	15	7.7	1.03
tofu curd	1/4 of a block	7	3.5	0.5
tofu	125 ml/1/2 c	11	5.5	0.7
almonds	30 g/1 oz	15	3.1	0.11
peanuts	30 g/1 oz	14	4.4	traces
walnuts	30 g/1 oz	16	9.5	0.94
pine nuts	30 g/1 oz	17	7.1	0.22
pistachio nuts	30 g/1 oz	15	2.2	0.08
sunflower seeds	15 ml/1 tbsp	4	2.8	0.01
MILK, MILK PRODUCTS,/ and SOY MILK				
cheddar cheese	30 g/1 oz	10.8	0.1	0.13
swiss cheese	30 g/1 oz	7.8	0.2	0.1
whole milk	250 ml/1 c	8.6	0.2	0.19
soy milk	250 ml/1 c	4.6	1.8	0.24

As you can see, whole grains and cereal products supply very little fat, but do contain proportionately more essential fatty acids than meat or dairy products. Oils and nuts supply large amounts of fat and large amounts of the essential fatty acids. Soybeans are very rich in essential fatty acids, and exceptionally rich in alpha-linolenic acid. Fruits and vegetables contain very little fat but proportionately more alpha-linolenic acid than many other foods. Soy milk contains less fat than whole milk but a good proportion of linoleic and alpha-linolenic acids.

If you add up the two essential fatty acids (the two last columns on the right) in a particular food, you will find that the sum never equals the total amount of fat for that food. This is not a trick or a mathematical error. Foods normally contain many different fatty acids that are not necessarily essential and are not listed in the chart. For example, 60 milliliters (4 tbsp) of wheat germ contains 1.71 grams of essential fatty acids and a total fat content of 2.8 grams, so there is a small amount of other fatty acids in wheat germ; 250 milliliters (1 cup) of whole milk contains 0.39 gram of essential fatty acids for a total fat content of 8.6 grams, so there is a fair amount of other fatty acids in whole milk. This is only part of the story of fatty acids in each food, but it underlines the importance of choosing the right quality of fats in a complete diet.

> *Even though their contribution is vital, essential fatty acids represent only a small part of the fats we eat. There is no benefit in eating large amounts.*

2

For Worse...

Although cholesterolphobia has surely been taken to extremes, present-day levels of fat consumption cannot be ignored. When an individual has a family history of degenerative diseases and consumes loads of bad fat, he multiplies his risk of developing heart disease, cancer, and autoimmune disease. He may also become obese and therefore compound his risks even further.

Cardiovascular disease

At the present time 40 million Americans have been diagnosed with cardiovascular disease, 80 million have elevated cholesterol levels, and 1.5 million die each year of heart attacks. More Canadian men and women die of heart disease and stroke each year than of any other illness. Approximately one out of four Canadians has some form of heart disease, and 40 percent of deaths caused by cardiovascular diseases are directly linked to high blood cholesterol.

In Ontario, 42 percent of adults have a total blood cholesterol level above the desired 5.2 mmol/L. In French Canada, where there have been many marriages within families and little mobility, heart disease can be related to genetic deficiencies. Such deficiencies could explain the 63 percent incidence of high blood cholesterol levels among Quebecers, say Dr. Jean Davignon, medical researcher at the Clinical Research Institute of Montreal, and his colleagues at the Center for Science and Health at the University of Dallas.

Our comprehension of the cholesterol and heart disease connection made headway thanks to a series of studies carried out in

Framingham, a small New England town. For nearly thirty years, doctors followed every single individual in that locality. The information they gathered allowed them to establish a definite link between the blood cholesterol level of an individual and his risk of developing heart disease. Their conclusions are clear: the higher the blood cholesterol level, the greater the risk.

But be careful. It is not necessarily the cholesterol found in food that has the greatest influence on the cholesterol in blood. Animal fats can share part of the blame as can highly processed fats. More and more research is now paying attention to the possible links between highly processed fats and cardiovascular disease, and is looking more closely at the impact of hydrogenation, an industrial process that triggers the formation of *trans*-fatty acids (see chapter 4). But again, the fats we eat cannot take all the blame. Our lifestyle, lack of physical activity, excess stress, and use of tobacco also play determinant roles.

Still, one thing remains certain: the more animal fats and processed fats a population eats, the greater the incidence of cardiovascular disease.

In the fifties, the Japanese consumed very little visible fat and very little meat; their incidence of cardiovascular disease was among the lowest in the world. Forty years later, the Japanese are eating more meat and using more processed fats; their consumption of total fat has quadrupled, and death from cardiovascular disease has more than tripled. Even though the incidence of cardiovascular disease in Japan remains among the lowest in the industrialized nations, this major shift in the quality and quantity of fat intake has been associated with a much higher incidence of infarction.

In the seventies, a group of Danish investigators compared the incidence of sudden death from cardiovascular disease in Danes with that in Greenland Inuit. They found that the death rate for the Inuit was significantly lower even though their diet was high in fat, even higher than that of the Danes. The difference was in the *type* of fat eaten by the Inuit rather than the quantity; their diet of fish and marine mammals contained five times more omega-3 fatty acids than the Danish diet.

More recently, a well-publicized study carried out by Dr. Walter Willet and a team of scientists at Harvard University also discussed the impact of the type of fat we eat. These researchers followed more than 80,000 nurses for eight years (from 1980 to 1988), monitored their food and fat intake on a regular basis, and noted all cardiovascular accidents during this period. At the end of the study, they noticed that women who had consumed 20 milliliters (4 tsp) a day of hydrogenated margarine had a greater incidence of heart problems than those who had eaten less than 5 milliliters (1 tsp). The risk increased as the consumption of cookies and refined bakery products prepared with hydrogenated fat increased. This team of Harvard scientists concluded that the higher the intake of hydrogenated fats, the higher the risk of cardiovascular problems in this female population. They added that it was not the total quantity of fat that made the difference, but rather the kind of fat, in this case, hydrogenated fat.

Another study conducted at six Boston hospitals by researchers at the Harvard School of Public Health looked at the effect of *trans*-fatty-acid intake (from processed fats) on coronary risk in both men and women. A total of 239 victims who survived their first heart attack and 282 healthy control subjects were questioned about the types of fat they used on bread, and in frying and baking. The increased risk was significant among those consuming more than 2.5 pats of margarine per day, and these findings support the hypothesis that links hydrogenated fats to heart disease.

At the Boston University Medical Center Hospital, Edward Siguel and Robert Lerman analyzed the fatty acids in the blood of confirmed cardiac patients and compared their results with those of healthy reference individuals. They found significantly more *trans*-fatty acids in the blood of the cardiac patients. As we saw earlier, the fatty acids in the blood are directly proportional to the fatty acids in the person's diet. The authors thus conclude that the consumption of hydrogenated fats and *trans*-fatty acids can now be considered a risk factor for heart disease.

In the editorial in the May 1994 issue of the *American Journal of Public Health*, Dr. Walter Willett reiterated the connection between hydrogenated fats and heart disease and estimated that, in the United States, 30,000 deaths per year could be associated with the consumption of hydrogenated fats.

These studies, which have measured fat intake and heart disease in different population groups, come to a common conclusion: it is the *type* of fat that makes the difference. Other studies, called clinical trials, have looked at diets to repair the damage in high-risk individuals. Until now, very few studies have shown a true reversal of heart disease.

Surgery was the classical recourse to clear up obstructed arteries until Dr. Dean Ornish, director of the Institute of Research in Preventive Medicine in Sausalito, California, made the news with his more healthful lifestyle approach. Dr. Ornish achieved a world first by showing that in only twelve months, a more healthful lifestyle could regress artery lesions in seriously ill cardiac patients, *without surgery or cholesterol-lowering drugs*. He followed forty-one subjects divided into two groups; twenty-two made important changes in their diet, ate a vegetarian diet with very little fat (less than 10 percent of the calories consumed in a day), increased their physical activity, and worked on different strategies when dealing with stress; the nineteen others (the control group) followed the usual recommendation of a diet containing 30 percent fat, and some aerobic exercise. No one smoked.

At the beginning of the program, Dr. Ornish took photographs of the interiors of the arteries of all patients (a procedure called angiography); after twelve months, he repeated the examination and saw that the blockages had regressed in the arteries of the first group of people but had increased slightly in the control group. Four years later, arteries continue to clear up in those who continued the more healthful lifestyle. Dr. Ornish's program does not guarantee positive results, but it demonstrates that a more healthful lifestyle can help a majority of patients. The very significant reduction in animal and processed fat and the shift toward foods rich in both essential fatty acids (whole grains and soy-based foods) has had spectacular effects on blocked arteries.

While there is significant research linking cardiovascular disease to a diet rich in animal fat and, more recently, to highly processed fats, no study has ever shown that maintaining the status quo, that is, continuing our present diet and lifestyle, will reverse or improve the chances of heart disease.

Cancer

In Canada, cancer is the second cause of death, after heart disease. Colon and rectal cancer cause 6,300 deaths per year, while breast cancer strikes one Canadian woman in eleven; 121,000 new cases of cancer are diagnosed each year, and more than 61,000 deaths are reported in Canadian cancer statistics. From 1981 to 1988, the incidence of all cancers combined increased by an annual average of 0.8 percent in men and 0.5 percent in women. Not too reassuring.

During the past twenty-five years, studies carried out in different countries have linked environmental factors to about 90 percent of all cancers. Researchers link diet to 35 percent of all cases, but research does not yet identify which foods or substances are carcinogenic for everyone, all the time. Age, heredity, and hormonal factors are among the numerous other puzzle pieces that must be taken into consideration before definite conclusions can be reached.

The connection between diet and cancer has preoccupied people for a very long time. However, it was only at the beginning of the twentieth century that researchers noted that undernourished laboratory rats had fewer cancerous tumors than rats fed abundantly. Not until the thirties and forties did we note other dietary changes that could influence the appearance of cancer in animals. For example, mammary tumors increased in number when rats were given more fat in their diet.

At the same time, researchers in epidemiology, the science that evaluates the frequency and causes of diseases in populations, had observed that the number of cases and types of cancer varied considerably from one region of the world to another, from one cultural group to another.

In the mid-seventies, epidemiological studies on **breast cancer** incidence revealed that this type of cancer was less frequent in developing countries and Japan, but that the incidence increased when individuals emigrated from these countries to the United States. For example, Japanese people living in Japan consume four times less fat and eat different fats than Americans, and have four times less the incidence of breast cancer. The incidence grows gradually when they immigrate to the United States, and approaches little by little that of native Americans. Another example is found in Israel where Jewish women coming from Asia and Africa have a lower incidence of breast cancer than those who come from Europe, thanks in part to a previous diet that contained less fat.

Researchers under the direction of Dr. Jacques Brisson of Laval University in Quebec City evaluated the diets of 640 women with breast cancer. Their analysis of all mammograms indicates that the damage was more limited in women who ate less fat of animal origin.

Another study conducted in Australia and published in 1990 shows that a diet rich in animal fat is associated with higher blood concentration of prolactin, and that a high level of prolactin is known to increase the risk of breast cancer in premenopausal women.

In general, the incidence of breast cancer rises with the increased consumption of fat, while the survival rate increases when the diet is poor in fat. An example of the second trend is taken from a study done in Asia in which postmenopausal Japanese women with breast cancer live ten years longer than American women in similar circumstances.

Colon cancer provides another model almost identical to breast cancer but seems even more closely associated with a diet rich in fat. High intakes of fat increase the amounts of fatty acids and bile acids in the colon, irritate the colonic cells, and act as tumor-promoting agents, which in turn induce cancer. Although this disease is rare in developing countries and Japan, it is found more frequently in emigrants from these countries living in the United States and in other industrialized countries.

Researchers from Harvard University under the direction of Dr. Walter Willet studied the effect of meat, fat, and fiber on colon cancer. They analyzed, by means of a questionnaire, the dietary habits of more than 80,000 women, and followed them closely for six years. According to their data, women who ate more red meat were twice as vulnerable to colon cancer compared with those who ate white meat and fish. It must be mentioned, however, that women who ate red meat also consumed more of all fats.

A similar study conducted in the Netherlands found after three and a half years that processed meats (not fresh meats) were associated with a higher risk of colon cancer in both sexes.

Skin cancer has attracted much attention in recent years, but the fat connection has seldom been researched. To fill the void, Homer Black and his fellow workers in Houston recently evaluated the impact of a lower fat intake on the incidence of sun-induced skin damage. For twenty-four months, they followed seventy-six patients with a history of nonmelanoma skin cancer and assigned half of them to a lower-fat diet (20 percent of calories); after two years, patients on the low-fat diet had a reduced incidence of the this form of skin tumor. "This effect can now be added to the list of potential benefits of a low-fat diet," concluded the authors.

Prostate cancer is the fourth most common site of cancer among men worldwide and causes over 4,000 deaths per year in Canada. Studies that compared prostate cancer rates among countries reveal substantial differences between the fat intake in areas with high incidence and those with low incidence. Other studies have looked at afflicted individuals and compared their diets with those of healthy individuals; ten out of thirteen studies show an evident association between fat, especially animal fat, and the risk of cancer. Loïc Le Marchand and his co-workers at the University of Hawaii evaluated the food consumption of over 20,000 men and followed these men between 1980 and 1989; their results published in *Epidemiology* in May 1994 indicate that a higher consumption of all meats and dairy products increased the risk of prostate cancer among these men.

The risk of **pancreatic cancer** can also be increased by the consumption of high-fat foods, such as sausages and bacon, says a study conducted in Utah involving 149 individuals with pancreatic cancer and 363 individuals in the general population.

Significant consumption of animal fat in particular has been incriminated in the development of many cancers, but animal fat cannot be entirely blamed. The classic studies done in the late seventies by Dr. Ken Carroll at the University of Western Ontario have clearly shown that diets rich in corn oil markedly increased the number of tumors in rats when compared with diets rich in animal fat. Excessive amounts of fats of vegetable origin can also increase our cells' vulnerability to certain cancers.

Other diseases of the immune system, such as diabetes, Crohn's disease, lupus, and rheumatoid arthritis, affect from 5 to 7 percent of the population; those who suffer from these problems seem to become allergic to certain constituents of their own body.

Food has an influence on the immune system. It must supply sufficient proteins, vitamins, minerals, and essential fatty acids to satisfy our needs. When in adequate supply, these nutrients reinforce the system. When in short supply, our defense mechanisms are weakened. Inadequacies usually affect the most vulnerable groups, young children and the elderly.

According to current knowledge, some foods rich in certain types of fat seem to play a more specific role. Lowering our fat intake can improve our immune system. Selecting the right type of fat is another powerful strategy. As we saw in chapter 1, fats rich in omega-3 fatty acids, such as linseed and fish oil, have been the object of several experimental and clinical studies and have demonstrated their beneficial action on the immune system. Hydrogenated fats have been shown to alter the immune system in mice; studies on humans are yet to come.

> *Always remember that large quantities of any fat can harm the immune system.*

Weight problems

In our society, obesity is an important, delicate, and controversial issue that leads to people spending billions of dollars each year on diets, diet products, and health care.

In Canada, 26 to 39 percent of adults older than twenty and from 5 to 25 percent of children are obese. In the United States, preliminary information from the latest health survey indicates that the problem is getting worse. North Americans are becoming heavier and heavier but surely not healthier. Cardiovascular disease, hypertension, diabetes, back pain, knee pain, and low self-esteem are all side effects that affect obese people to a larger or smaller degree. Obesity can even impair the immune system and increase the risk of certain cancers.

Obesity means weighing at least 20 percent more than one's healthy weight and is quite different from carrying a few extra pounds. In other words, being pleasantly plump is not a health problem — even if weighing ten extra pounds has ruined too many lives and counting calories has spoiled too many meals. Diets are now at a major turning point; cutting calories per se is no longer the correct answer to losing weight. Current research links fat to obesity and is opening bright new perspectives.

First of all, researchers have noticed that heavy individuals have a higher fat intake than lean individuals even if they have the same calorie intake. Fat people consume at least 35 percent of their calories in the form of fat and 46 percent of their calories in the form of carbohydrates; slimmer people consume 29 percent of their calories in the form of fat and 53 percent in the form of carbohydrates. They also noted that the slim are physically more active than fat individuals. It is not the quantity of *calories* that make the difference but the quantity of *fat* and *physical activity*. This observation has also been made in China, where the Chinese consume more calories but much less fat than we do, and rarely suffer weight problems.

At a recent conference of the American Dietetic Association, S. McKinney and P. Buccacio of Drexel University in Philadelphia confirmed the theory that excessive fat intake is the main cause of weight problems. They emphasized that the *source* of calories seems to be more important than the total amount of calories. Thus, a diet rich in cereal products, bread, beans and pasta, lean dairy products, fruits, and vegetables and poor in fat could favor weight loss without counting calories.

Then researchers tested the hypothesis. They conducted a study over a period of six months with premenopausal women to see if the risk of heart disease could be reduced by cutting down the amount of fat to 20 percent of the daily calories. Even though they consumed the same amount of calories and had the same level of physical activity as the control group, these women lost weight and fat tissue. Another study carried out over two years with 300 menopausal women arrived at the same conclusion: a significant reduction in dietary fat without a significant reduction of calories produces weight loss.

Scientists have more than one explanation for this unexpected reaction. Klaas Westerstep of the University of Limburg in the Netherlands explains it as being the result of the body's greater ability to burn proteins and carbohydrates than to burn fat. In fact, the body's normal reaction is to store fat for future use. David Pan and Leonard Storlien of the Garvan Institute of Medical Research in Australia looked at the fate of different types of fats; they tested the impact on weight gain of three high-fat diets with a similar calorie content on laboratory rats; the rats fed the diet with a higher omega-3 fatty-acid content gained less weight than did the others. George Mann of Nashville, Tennessee, has been seriously questioning the impact of hydrogenated fats and suggests that *trans*-fatty acids (from hydrogenated fats) may impair the retrieval of fat from fat cells.

At our nutrition clinic, we have never believed in the effectiveness of calorie-reduced diets, and for many years we have had an antidiet approach. Since research on the benefits of fat reduction emerged, we developed a new eating strategy based on a low-fat approach. The response has been most enthusiastic, especially among ex-dieters. Guilt-free plates filled with pasta, slices of whole-wheat bread, generous servings of brown rice, fruit, and vegetables, and adequate amounts of low-fat milk products make for much happier dieters. Weight loss is achieved in many cases, especially when regular physical activity is included.

> *While permanent weight loss can only be achieved if lifestyle changes are maintained, changes in lifestyle alone cannot solve weight problems. Both the quality and the quantity of fats consumed can have a major impact on obesity.*

3

The Cholesterol Saga

Should we worry about the cholesterol in shrimps? What is a high blood cholesterol level? Is the cholesterol in an egg "good" cholesterol? Is a "cholesterol free" salad dressing more healthful than olive oil and vinegar? So many questions and so much confusion surround this critical topic

Cholesterol is naturally present in everybody's blood and in many foods. But let's not mix *blood* cholesterol with *dietary* cholesterol.

Blood cholesterol

Blood cholesterol is a fatty substance that travels normally in the blood to carry out different tasks in the body. But a fatty substance needs help to travel in a watery liquid such as blood. Cholesterol therefore requires a special transportation system and uses proteins that specialize in fat transportation in the blood. These substances are called *lipoproteins*. The most talked about are low-density lipoproteins, or LDL, and high-density lipoproteins, or HDL.

The LDL pick up the cholesterol in the liver, our main production site, and transport it to cells elsewhere in the body. When the quantity of cholesterol transported by LDL is excessive, the overload sticks to the lining of the arteries and gradually narrows the arteries until the blood can no longer flow through them. If the affected arteries are coronary arteries, a heart attack follows. For this reason, LDL do not have a good reputation and are labeled "bad cholesterol."

The HDL are responsible for the return journey. They pick up excess cholesterol in the blood and cells; they can even gather some of the cholesterol stuck to the arteries and bring it all back to the liver, which then eliminates the cholesterol load with the help of bile. Because of their cleansing action, the HDL are called "good cholesterol."

Apolipoproteins A1 and Apolipoproteins B, which travel along with the HDL and LDL, are tiny particles that recognize the sites where they can deposit their cargo of cholesterol. Apo-A1 travel on HDL or "good cholesterol," and Apo-B travel on LDL or "bad cholesterol."

Formerly, blood analyses gave only the total amount of cholesterol in the blood. Today, analyses can specify the amounts of good cholesterol (HDL) and bad cholesterol (LDL). Certain laboratories use more accurate methods and measure the levels of Apo-A1 and Apo-B.

The initial blood test will usually measure total cholesterol only. When the total cholesterol exceeds the norm of 5.2 mmol/L, a second blood test is recommended to measure the lipoproteins HDL and LDL. If the LDL (bad cholesterol) exceed 4.25 mmol/L while the HDL (good cholesterol) are below 1 mmol/L, there is a problem. If, on the other hand, the HDL (good cholesterol) is high (more than 2 mmol/L) and the ratio between total cholesterol and HDL is equal to or lower than 4.5, the likelihood of cardiovascular problems is slim.

For example, Mr. Martin, sixty-five years old, has a normal weight but is quite inactive; his total cholesterol is 7.04, with an HDL of 1.16 and LDL of 5.19. The ratio between his total cholesterol and HDL is 6.06 compared with the recommended ratio of 4.5.

Mrs. Smith is sixty-three, with a healthy weight and a moderate level of activity. When she came to our clinic, her total cholesterol was 6.63, HDL of 0.50, LDL of 5.13. The ratio between her total cholesterol and her HDL was 13.2, which greatly exceeds the 4.5 ratio and is considered a high risk for heart disease. After modifying her diet with a *good fat, bad fat* approach for several months, her total cholesterol dropped to 5.94, her HDL increased to 2.3, and her LDL dropped to 3.23. The new ratio between the total cholesterol and HDL dropped to 2.58, which represents no risk of heart disease.

These examples illustrate the limited value of one total cholesterol figure because it is impossible to evaluate the risks without having the whole picture. It also shows that a nutritional approach can have a positive impact on the risk factor.

Table 2 summarizes blood values that are acceptable and at risk, at different ages. Consider all aspects of your last blood test and work toward maintaining a high HDL (good cholesterol) value. Write your blood values in the last column on the right and evaluate your risk factor.

AGE GROUP	MMOL/L	COMMENTS	YOUR LAST BLOOD TEST
Table 2			
Blood analysis			
Total cholesterol			
65 years or older	6.2 or less	acceptable	
30 to 65	5.2 or less	acceptable	
	6.2 or more	at risk	
18 to 29	4.6 or less	acceptable	
	5.7 or more	at risk	
HDL (good cholesterol)			
all age groups	1.1 or more	acceptable	
	0.9 or less	at risk	
LDL (bad cholesterol)			
65 years and older	4.1 or less	acceptable	
30 to 65	3.4 or less	acceptable	
	4.2 or more	at risk	
18 to 29	3.0 or less	acceptable	
Triglycerides			
all age groups	2.3 or less	acceptable	
Apo A1			
all age groups	1.07 to 1.35 g/L	acceptable	
Apo B			
all age groups	0.87 to 1.11 g/L	acceptable	
Apo A1/Apo B			
all age groups	1.07 to 1.53 g/L	acceptable	

This having been said, a recent study conducted with over 6,000 individuals in six different communities of Minnesota has shown that, in some cases, a low HDL (good cholesterol) is not associated with a high risk of heart disease, especially if the total cholesterol is within or below the normal range. The Ornish study, which has shown a real reversal of cardiac symptoms, concludes that lifestyle changes (very-low-fat diet, exercise, and relaxation) have a greater impact on coronary artery lesions than on blood cholesterol levels. In other words, such lifestyle changes can increase the blood flow in the coronary arteries and yet show minor reductions in blood cholesterol values.

> *So don't count on blood cholesterol values alone. Work on more than one front!*

While everyone worries about excess cholesterol in their blood, it is important to keep in mind that the human body cannot function properly without a certain amount of cholesterol. In fact, cholesterol is produced by the body itself; it can also be supplied by some of the food we eat. Whatever the source, cholesterol is used for several important jobs, such as the proper functioning of the brain and the production of certain hormones and of vitamin D. The body has such a need for cholesterol that it is available in mother's milk, even if the mother never consumes cholesterol in her food.

Triglycerides, another fatty substance that travels in the blood, have a tendency to increase when there is an excess of alcohol, fat, and sweets in the diet. Although triglycerides are not considered to be as important a risk factor as high levels of LDL (bad cholesterol), it seems desirable to normalize blood values at a level below 2.3 mmol/L.

Cholesterol in food

In contrast to the essential fatty acids, which need to be supplied by the diet, cholesterol is not an essential nutrient because the body can manufacture enough of it on its own. That is why a diet without any food cholesterol never triggers a cholesterol deficiency. For that matter, there is no *good* and no *bad* cholesterol in food, nor is there any HDL or LDL in foods.

Only animals can produce cholesterol; only foods of animal origin contain cholesterol. Liver, kidneys, eggs, and caviar contain lots of it, while meat, fowl, and dairy products contain less. Foods of plant origin, including vegetable oils, almonds, nuts, seeds, olives, cereal products, and dried legumes, fruits, and vegetables contain no trace of cholesterol. The division is as clean and clear as that!

Table 3 lists animal foods that contain very little fat but a lot of cholesterol; Table 4 lists plant foods that are rich in fat but contain no trace of cholesterol.

Table 3			
Foods *low in fat* but *rich in cholesterol*			
FOOD	PORTION	FAT (g)	CHOLESTEROL (mg)
shrimps	100 g/3 oz	1.1	150
crab	100 g/3 oz	1.9	100
sweetbreads	100 g/3 oz	3.2	466
chicken liver	100 g/3 oz	5.5	631

Table 4			
Foods *rich in fat* but *cholesterol free*			
FOOD	PORTION	FAT (g)	CHOLESTEROL (mg)
oil	15 ml/1 tbsp	14	0
avocado	half	15	0
peanut butter	30 ml/2 tbsp	18	0
chips	small bag	21	0
mixed nuts	75 ml/5 tbsp	28	0

Remember, it is not necessarily cholesterol-rich foods that have the greatest impact on blood cholesterol levels.

4

Different Fats in Different Foods

When you read the labels on food products, you become acquainted with the fat jargon, which includes such terms as *saturated, polyunsaturated,* and *monounsaturated.* These terms correspond to three types of fatty acids with unique characteristics, properties, and behavior in the body. To complicate the issue, a food naturally contains more than one type of fatty acid.

When we digest meat, olive oil, or butter, we gradually transform the dietary fat into usable fatty acids. These fatty acids are substances that present themselves as long, medium, or short chains. Picture fatty acids as bracelets with metal links, each link coupled to its two neighboring links and able to receive two charms, one on each side of the link (see Figure 1).

The foods we eat contain different proportions of saturated, monounsaturated, and polyunsaturated fatty acids. Meats and dairy products contain a high proportion of saturated fatty acids; almonds and olives have a higher proportion of monounsaturated fatty acids; sunflower oil and corn oil contain significant proportions of polyunsaturated fatty acids. Usually, a food rich in saturated fat is solid at room temperature, while a food rich in mono- or polyunsaturated fat is liquid. The more of one type of fatty acid a food contains, the more it adopts the behavior of this predominant fatty acid.

The saturated fats

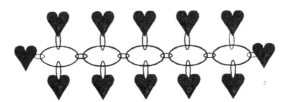

Figure 1: A saturated fatty-acid chain

As illustrated in Figure 1, a saturated fatty acid is rigid, like a ruler. Each link of the bracelet has its full complement of two charms and cannot take any additional charms.

Saturated fatty acids have a tendency to raise the blood cholesterol level in vulnerable individuals, but not all saturated fats behave alike. The saturated fatty acid found in butter and dairy foods dramatically raises the LDL (bad cholesterol) while the one found in beef increases LDL to a lesser degree, and the one in cocoa butter has an even smaller impact.

Saturated fatty acids are found mainly in fats of animal origin such as meat and dairy products, but certain plant foods like palm oil and coconut oil are exceptions to the rule and also contain large amounts (see page 90).

A certain amount of saturated fats can be eaten in a healthful diet, but a significant intake leads to trouble. As shown in Table 5, foods rich in saturated fats also contain other types of fat.

Table 5 Foods rich in saturated fatty acids					
FOOD	PORTION	FAT (g)	SATURATED (g)	MONO (g)	POLY (g)
Camembert	30 g/1 oz	7	4.3	2.0	0.2
whole milk	250 ml/1 cup	9	5.1	2.4	0.4
butter	10 ml/2 tsp	8	5.0	2.3	0.3
coconut	125 ml/1/2 cup	13	12.4	0.6	0.2

The monounsaturated fats

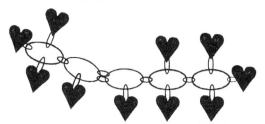

Figure 2: A monounsaturated fatty-acid chain

As illustrated, the chain of a monounsaturated fatty acid is slightly curved and has only one double link that can receive two additional charms.

Until recently the impact of monounsaturated fatty acids on cholesterol was virtually unknown. Modern research, more accurate blood tests, and mid-eighties studies on the Mediterranean diet, which is rich in olive oil, a monounsaturated fat, changed the whole picture. We now know that monounsaturated fats can reduce the total cholesterol and the LDL while protecting the HDL, the good cholesterol. A diet rich in monounsaturated fats can also lower triglycerides, the other fatty substance in the blood. Research done on diabetics shows that monounsaturated fatty acids improve the control of blood sugar and can significantly reduce daily insulin requirements.

Monounsaturated fats are found in plant foods such as olive oil, canola oil, hazelnut oil, almonds, avocados, pistachios, and macadamia nuts. A significant intake of such foods will not increase your risk of heart disease but can promote weight gain.

As shown in Table 6, foods rich in monounsaturated fats also contain small amounts of saturated and polyunsaturated fats.

Table 6 Foods rich in monounsaturated fatty acids					
FOOD	PORTION	FAT (g)	SATURATED (g)	MONO (g)	POLY (g)
salmon	100 g/3 oz	11	3.2	5.0	3.1
olive oil	15 ml/1 tbsp	13	1.8	9.9	1.2
pistachio	75 ml/5 tbsp	18	2.3	12.5	2.8
almonds	75 ml/5 tbsp	21	2.1	14.4	4.2
avocado	1 half	15	2.2	9.7	1.8

The polyunsaturated fats

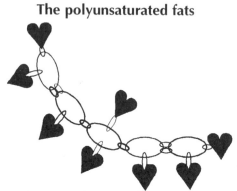

Figure 3: A polyunsaturated fatty-acid chain

As Figure 3 illustrates, the polyunsaturated fatty-acid chain is definitely more curved than other fatty acids. It can incorporate at least four new charms by reorganizing the two double links. The more double links in a fatty acid, the greater the instability and risk of oxidation.

Polyunsaturated fatty acids have long been the most promoted by health professionals because of their rich content in essential fatty acids and because of their power to reduce total blood cholesterol. But since blood tests have become more accurate, scientists have noticed that while polyunsaturated fatty acids lowered total cholesterol and the LDL (bad cholesterol), they could lower the HDL (good cholesterol), which is a serious drawback. Research has also demonstrated that a diet rich in polyunsaturated fats can promote tumor growth in animal species.

As mentioned previously, oxidation is not uncommon in foods rich in polyunsaturated fats; it alters the flavor of the food, which becomes rancid, sharp, and unpleasant.

In the human body, oxidation is a natural process that promotes energy production, but oxidation also plays a role in the formation of toxic substances called free radicals. In our bodies, oxidized polyunsaturated fatty acids called peroxides become incapable of doing their jobs in the cellular membrane. Foods rich in polyunsaturated fats usually have a natural shield, vitamin E, which protects the fatty acid and the cell from this oxidation, but processing destroys part of this useful vitamin.

Polyunsaturated fatty acids are found in plant foods such as corn, soya, wheat germ, safflower, sunflower, and sesame-seed oils, as well as sunflower and sesame seeds.

As shown in Table 7, foods rich in polyunsaturated fatty acids also contain small amounts of other types of fat.

Table 7 Foods rich in polyunsaturated fats from the omega-6 family					
FOOD	PORTION	FAT	SATURATED	MONO	POLY
		(g)	(g)	(g)	(g)
soya oil	15 ml/1 tbsp	14	2.0	3.2	7.8
sunflower oil	15 ml/1 tbsp	14	1.4	2.7	8.9
corn oil	15 ml/1 tbsp	14	1.7	3.3	8.0
sesame seeds	75 ml/5 tbsp	21	3.0	9.0	9.0

The family of polyunsaturated fatty acids is a very large family that includes both the omega-6 and the omega-3 fatty acids. The omega-3 fatty acids, discussed in greater detail in chapter 1, can lower triglycerides and protect the HDL (good cholesterol). They can retard the formation of blood clots in the arteries, have a beneficial action on arterial blood pressure, and seem to play an anti-inflammatory, anti-tumor role in many cases. Omega-3 fatty acids are found mainly in fish, especially fatty fish, but also in linseed oil, canola oil, walnuts, soybeans, and some dark green leafy vegetables.

Table 8 Foods rich in polyunsaturated fats from the omega-3 family			
FOOD	PORTION	FAT (g)	OMEGA-3 (g)
salmon	100 g/3 oz	11.0	2.0
mackerel	100 g/3 oz	14.0	3.1
linseed oil	5 ml/1 tsp	4.5	2.4
walnuts	75 ml/5 tbsp	22.0	2.5
spinach	250 ml/1 cup	0.5	0.2
purslane	250 ml/1 cup	0.3	0.2
broccoli	250 ml/1 cup	0.2	0.1
soybeans	250 ml/1 cup	15.0	1.0

Hydrogenated fats and *trans*-fatty acids

The preceding fatty acids have been present in our foods since the Garden of Eden. But relatively recently, the food industry has seriously modified the most vulnerable among them, the poly- and monounsaturated fatty acids, in order to obtain a solid and stable fat at room temperature. Chemists and food technologists have developed a very effective method called *hydrogenation*. Large quantities of oil are heated in a vacuum; once the proper temperature is reached, hydrogen is forced under pressure into the oil. The mixture is whipped until the desired amount of hydrogen is incorporated into the fatty acids. This addition of hydrogen to the fatty acid makes it a *hydrogenated* fatty acid.

Hydrogenation is a well-recognized and common industrial process. It raises the melting point of a fat, hardens and stabilizes it. It extends storage time and permits the use of higher cooking temperatures. It is very useful from an industrial point of view but less useful for our bodies. When oils are hydrogenated, their unsaturated fatty acids lose their natural form, called *cis*, and assume a new form called *trans*, a sort of nonidentical twin with different characteristics altogether.

This chemical shift into the *trans* form changes the entire behavior of the unsaturated fatty acids. Instead of acting normally, they act much like saturated fats: they increase the LDL (bad cholesterol), decrease the HDL (good cholesterol), and increase the risk of heart disease. On the whole, they compete with essential fatty acids and may lead to a deficiency, which can affect the arteries and the immune system. They produce derivatives that do not function like the original prostaglandins (see chapter 1) and have a negative impact on cell-membrane fluidity and behavior.

The list of the possible adverse effects of *trans*-fatty acids was recently lengthened to include complications with diabetes and weight problems. Researchers are also looking at the connection with cancer, but no one has yet found conclusive evidence that this seriously modified fat is a factor in the development of cancers.

Meanwhile, hydrogenated fats and *trans*-fatty acids are found in a wide range of food products.

A series of analyses done by the Bureau of Nutritional Sciences at Health and Welfare Canada in 1993 looked at the fatty acids in seventeen food categories sold in the Canadian retail market; one hundred common food items were analyzed, and it was found that:

- One slice of **bread** contains approximately 0.1 gram of *trans*-fatty acids.
- One **hamburger bun** contains approximately 0.8 gram of *trans*-fatty acids.
- One piece of **cake** contains between 1 and 3 grams of *trans*-fatty acids.
- A few **candies** or a **chocolate bar** contain approximately 0.9 gram of *trans*-fatty acids.
- A bowl of **cereal** contains from 0.2 to 0.7 gram of *trans*-fatty acids.
- One **cookie** contains from 0.3 to 2 grams of *trans*-fatty acids.
- A **cracker** contains from 0.4 to 1 gram of *trans*-fatty acids.
- A **doughnut** contains from 2.8 to 3.3 grams of *trans*-fatty acids.
- A small portion of **french fries** (precooked) contains 1.3 to 1.7 grams of *trans*-fatty acids.
- A commercial **muffin** contains from 1.1 to 1.7 grams of *trans*-fatty acids.
- The **crust** of a medium slice of pizza contains 0.6 to 0.8 gram of *trans*-fatty acids.
- 15 ml or one tablespoon of **shortening** contains 2.2 to 2.6 grams of *trans*-fatty acids.
- A small bag of **potato chips** contains 7 to 9 grams of *trans*-fatty acids.
- A small bag of **corn chips** contains 5.7 to 6.5 grams of *trans*-fatty acids.

Another study on fifty brands of margarine sold in Canada revealed that in 1991, **stick (solid)** margarines contained from 26 to 50 percent *trans*-fatty acids while **tub (soft)** margarines had from 0 to 36 percent *trans*-fatty acids.

An individual who consumes margarine, cookies, crackers, and chips on a daily basis can easily ingest more than 10 grams of *trans*-fatty acids per day, a dose considered a health risk by some scientists.

Unfortunately, it is impossible for the consumer to detect the exact amounts of *trans*-fatty acids found in our foods, because federal laws and regulations do not require this type of information to appear on labels. The only indication we have is in the list of ingredients; the presence of any type of hydrogenated oil or shortening tells us that the food contains some *trans*-fatty acids.

> *There is much more to the cholesterol saga than watching the amount of cholesterol in individual foods. All the different fats in our foods affect our cells and our arteries — for better or for worse.*

5

Quality — the First Priority

Men and women have included some fat in their diet since the beginning of time, and we have no intention of changing that food habit. But before we give you our new golden rule, let's look at the spectacular changes that have taken place in the type and quantities of fat we eat.

The first fragment of information comes from prehistoric times, thanks to the work of American anthropologists who have studied the types of foods consumed 25,000 years ago. According to their findings, prehistoric humans ate a variety of game and fish, which were much leaner and lower in saturated fats than our present meat supply, but richer in polyunsaturated fatty acids and omega-3 fatty acids, and in some cholesterol. They also ate roots, leguminous plants (beans, peas, etc), nuts, tubers, and wild fruits, foods that are rich in fiber, vitamin C, and minerals. Thus, cavemen and women ate less fat than we do (about 20 percent of daily calories), but fat of good quality.

Cereal agriculture, beginning 10,000 years B.C., changed the food habits of humans by increasing the fiber content and reducing the proportion of fat to 15 percent of daily calories. Then olive oil made its appearance on the shores of the Mediterranean about 5,000 years ago; butter settled in a little later in the cooking of the Vikings and Normans. These foods were considered precious foods, consumed in small quantities and kept for special occasions. Remember Little Red Riding Hood walking through the forest with a little pot of butter for her grandmother? An unthinkable gift today. By the end of the nineteenth century, our great-grandparents were eating pork and beans, meat pies, stew, and pot roast, but not every day.

Since then, our food habits have deteriorated, especially in industrialized countries. With few exceptions, populations that have become wealthier have eaten more and more fat. The more industrialized they have become, the more they have consumed hydrogenated fats and fried foods. In short, *bad* fat.

For several reasons, the consumption of fats gradually but markedly changed. The daily diet included two instead of one main meal with meat, potatoes, gravy, and numerous slices of buttered bread. Then the food industry discovered how to stabilize oils by refining and hydrogenating them. The consumer learned to cook with margarine, bake with shortening, and ignore salad oil; he slowly developed a taste for fried and processed foods cooked by others. The status of fats slowly passed from that of a precious food eaten in small quantities to that of a nuisance, present in every dish, sticking to our arteries and expanding our waistlines.

After thirty-odd years of eating these new hydrogenated fats and larger servings of meat, eggs, and bacon, deaths from cardiovascular disease reached their peak. By the early sixties, scientists began to consider the relationship between different fats and modern diseases.

In recent years:

- Our daily intake of fat has increased from 25 percent to 40 percent of daily calories.
- Animal fats have slowly been replaced by hydrogenated vegetable oils.
- Margarine has replaced butter in many households.
- *Trans*-fatty acids have slipped into most margarines, crackers, cookies, french fries, and peanut butters.
- Fried foods are at the heart of most fast-foods meals.

In 1983, Canadians as well as Americans and Europeans ate more fat — and more bad fat — than ever, reaching more than 40 percent of daily calories, an all-time record. In 1990, more than 50 percent of all vegetable oil used in Canada was hydrogenated. In 1993, the fat composition of one hundred common items in seventeen food categories sold on the Canadian retail market was analyzed by scientists of the Nutrition Research Division of Health Canada. Of these items, fifty-two contained *trans*-fatty acids; breads, hamburger buns, cakes, candies, chocolate, doughnuts, french fries, muffins, pizza crusts, shortenings, popato chips, and corn chips all contained some (see chapter 4). Ashima Kant, a dietitian and researcher at the City University of New York, looked at the impact on our diet of "other foods" not listed in the Food Pyramid (the American version of Canada's Food Guide); she noted that foods low in nutrients but high in sugar and fat accounted for 30 percent of the daily calories and 30 percent of total fat intake. Cakes, cookies, pies, and crackers are filling us with bad fat. Health surveys indicate a recent reduction in our total fat intake, but Santé Québec, a health survey released in 1993, identified soft margarine as one of the main sources of fat in our diet.

Current statistics indicate that the daily fat intake is between 70 and 80 grams for a woman eating between 1,600 and 2,000 calories per day and 105 grams for a man who eats 2,500 calories per day (see the tables in the Appendix to convert grams of fat in foods). Our present fat intake is a problem because:

- It exceeds the intake recommended by the experts, which has been set at 30 percent of daily calories, and contains a fair amount of *bad* fat.
- Most importantly, this intake of *bad* fat competes with the essential fatty acids and their vital work at the cellular level.

Current recommendations and their limitations

Current recommendations invite us to decrease our excessive fat intake, but they seldom discuss our basic needs for essential fatty acids. The World Health Organization, the Canadian Cancer Society, the American Heart Association, the Heart and Stroke Foundation, and the National Cancer Institute are unanimous: the desirable fat intake is around 30 percent of daily calories. Health and Welfare Canada decreed in 1990 that the "diet of Canadians should not supply more than 30 percent of the total quantity of energy in the form of fat" toward the goal of reducing the incidence of cardiovascular disease and certain cancers. The practical suggestion is to eat different types of fats in equal quantities of saturates, monounsaturates, and polyunsaturates. In our opinion, this recommendation is still incomplete; it presents a confusing flurry of numbers without arousing distrust toward fats that are really harmful, and it doesn't lead to a concern for *quality*. First of all, "the 30 percent of calories" is an abstract figure that is poorly understood by consumers. Aimed at health professionals, this notion has bounced into the media, onto labels, and into advertising, but it spreads a lot of confusion. If consumers think that each food must respect the 30 percent fat limit, they may think they cannot even afford to eat such healthful foods as a real salad dressing, a few nuts, or slices of avocado. Such an interpretation falls short of the actual recommendation, which aims at reducing the *total quantity* of fat for the entire day, three meals and snacks included. Even within this context, the notion of 30 percent, to be suitably useful, involves several calculations and remains abstract.

Second, this recommendation attaches very little importance to the notion of the *quality* of fat. It suggests *"reducing total fat by choosing low-fat dairy products, lean meat, and foods prepared with little or no fat,"* but it gives no warning against fats that have been processed and hydrogenated and the *trans*-fatty acids, which increase the LDL (bad cholesterol) and lower the HDL (good cholesterol), affect the permeability of the cell membrane, and increase the risk of cardiovascular diseases. To speak of quantity of fat without stipulating the *quality* is nonsense. Past and recent research demonstrate that the *type* of fat has more impact on cardiovascular health than the 30 percent limit.

A study carried out in California on men and women with a high blood cholesterol level measured the importance of fat quality while increasing the total fat intake from 28 percent to 37 percent of daily calories. Gene Spiller and his colleagues replaced a good part of the saturated fat in the diet with monounsaturated fat from almonds and almond oil. Grains and cereal products, fruits, vegetables, legumes, nonfat or 2 percent fat dairy products, and fish were allowed in unlimited amounts. After nine weeks on the diet, total cholesterol and LDL (bad cholesterol) levels fell by 10 percent while HDL (good cholesterol) was maintained at the same level.

A similar study was conducted in Spain with women having no cholesterol problem. The researchers used three different types of fat; the first diet was rich in saturated fats, the second in polyunsaturates, and the third in monounsaturates. In spite of an increased fat intake to approximately 36 percent of calories in the three experimental diets, the third, based on olive oil, lowered total cholesterol levels as well as the LDL (bad cholesterol) and maintained a better proportion of HDL (good cholesterol) than the other two diets.

An Australian study compared the impact of a diet rich in carbohydrates and low in fat (20 percent of calories) with a diet richer in fat (36 percent of calories), but mainly monounsaturated fats. Fifteen healthy women between the ages of thirty-seven and fifty-eight saw their total cholesterol levels fall on the two diets. The diet rich in monounsaturated fats led to a significant drop in LDL (bad cholesterol) and the maintenance of HDL. On the other hand, the low-fat diet caused the HDL (good cholesterol) to fall by 13.9 percent. The authors of the study concluded that a diet rich in monounsaturated fat seems to be more efficient in reducing the risk of heart disease and the LDL (bad cholesterol) than a diet low in fat.

In Okinawa, a region of Japan where people live longer and where the incidence of cardiovascular diseases is lower than elsewhere in Japan, a study also showed that the *percentage* of fat in the diet is not always the most important factor. The Japanese of this region have a fat intake equivalent to 29 percent of their daily calories compared with 25 percent for Japan as a whole, but the authors point out that it is the ratio between the two essential fatty acids that makes the difference. The benefits seem to come from a higher proportion of foods rich in alpha-linolenic acid, the omega-3 family, than elsewhere in the country.

What shows up in all these studies related to cardiovascular-disease prevention is that the type of fat consumed has more impact than the 30 percent limit.

Third, even if the present recommendation is preferable to the current fat intake, the 30 percent limit does not suffice to clean out seriously blocked arteries. On the contrary! Dr. Ornish's studies showed that in high-risk patients, the 30 percent limit did not stop the narrowing of the arteries, while a major fat reduction to 10 percent of calories was shown to be efficient in cleaning up the arteries.

Dr. Colin Campbell of Cornell University coordinated the unique study called the China study, carried out in sixty-five cantons of the Republic of China. Teams of scientists compared the diets of the Chinese in different regions, took blood samples, and looked at the main causes of death. Having noted that the Chinese diet contains only 15 percent fat and that cardiovascular disease counts for only 1 percent of deaths, he has serious reservations as to the 30 percent norm for North Americans, which he bluntly considers a political norm. He also believes that to prevent various cancers, including breast cancer, the diet should contain more plant foods and fats should not exceed 20 percent of daily calories.

This third set of studies puts more emphasis on the benefits of lower fat intakes in specific cases, such as with high-risk cardiac patients or to prevent certain cancers. But even in the context of lower fat intake, it is the *quality* of the fat that is most important.

The French paradox

In all this debate about fats, the French find themselves in the middle of a scientific contradiction that experts call the *French paradox*: while the French consume just as much saturated fat as North Americans or as neighboring Europeans, they enjoy a lower incidence of death by cardiovascular disease.

The established connection between a high saturated-fat intake — and high blood cholesterol levels — and a heart attack at sixty does not apply to this population as it does to all the other industrialized countries.

Several teams of American and European researchers are attempting to solve the mystery by conducting various studies to compare the dietary habits of the French to those of other industrialized populations. Theories put forward for twenty-five years are suddenly giving way to a new hypothesis that is thrilling many people: red wine is thought to be beneficial, according to some experts. Reporters got their hands on this story in 1991, and it made the news while researchers were still researching. Since then, Dr. Serge Renaud of INSERM (Institut National de la Santé et de la Recherche Médicale) in France and his team of scientists have verified the protective action of red wine; according to this team, red wine has the power to inhibit the negative action of blood platelets, even after a very rich meal. In normal circumstances, the more saturated fats a meal contains the more the platelets reduce the blood's fluidity and the greater the risk of a heart attack. Another team of researchers in California measured the protective action of the polyphenols found in red wine; they concluded that polyphenols have an important antioxidant effect that can protect the lipoproteins in the blood, an even more powerful effect than that of vitamin E, a recognized antioxidant.

We compared the fat intake of the French at the beginning of the seventies to that of other industrialized countries and their neighbors; we found a net difference in the quality of fats consumed. While the Dutch ate 22 kilograms of margarine and shortening per year, the Swedes 18 kilograms, and the Germans and North Americans not less than 12 kilograms, the French consumed only butter and oil (see Table 9). The French have resisted margarine and other hydrogenated fats rich in *trans*-fatty acids much longer than have their fellow Europeans. We are not the only ones to have made this observation. George Mann also mentioned in 1994 that "the French paradox may be due to the limited use of partially hydrogenated fat in French foods."

The French have always indulged in good salad dressings made with olive oil rich in monounsaturated fats and walnut oil rich in omega-3 fatty acids, and in polyphenols and vitamin E, two antioxidants that are greatly reduced in refined oils. The French also enjoy fresh fish rich in omega-3 fatty acids and generous servings of various vegetables and fresh fruit. In short, they seem to know how to choose a better quality of fat.

Table 9 Individual fat intake (pounds/year), in 1975						
COUNTRY	TOTAL FAT	ANIMAL FAT		HYDROGENATED FAT		OILS
		butter	lard	margarine	shortening	
France	50.0	18.9	0.7	7.0	1.8	21.6
Germany	61.8	15.4	12.5	18.2	7.3	8.4
Japan	21.0	1.1	2.0	2.9	2.0	13.0
Netherlands	68.0	5.1	3.0	31.7	3.0	10.6
Sweden	57.4	11.7	0.9	38.5	0.9	3.7
UK	56.3	19.6	7.9	11.0	7.9	13.2
USA	53.7	4.8	3.1	10.8	3.1	17.6

Other aspects of their lifestyle, such as regular physical activity and time set aside for meals, may also contribute to the lower incidence of cardiovascular disease.

In our opinion, the notion of the *quality* of fat remains the crux of the matter.

Our basic needs

> *Our new golden rule: Give priority to quality.*

Giving priority to quality means finding the useful fats in our food supply. As we saw in chapter 1, every single cell in our body needs fat to function normally, but the kind of fat our cells need and the quantity they require no longer correspond with our present intake. To work well, our cells need the winning team of linoleic and alpha-linolenic acids, the two essential fatty acids; they expect them to function in a complementary fashion.

Compared to the current 75 or 100 grams of fat consumed each day, our real daily needs for essential fatty acids are quite minimal, vary little over the course of life, and are proportional to our calorie requirements. A growing adolescent needs more calories and a greater amount of essential fatty acids than an inactive elderly woman. These requirements are established by nutrition experts and are presented in the latest version of *Nutrition Recommendations for Canadians (1990)*. We actually need:

- From the omega-6 family: 7 to 11 grams of linoleic acid per day.
- From the omega-3 family: 1.1 to 1.8 grams of alpha-linolenic acid per day.

A ratio of 6 to 1 of linoleic acid to alpha-linolenic acid is recommended to maintain a healthy balance between the omega-6 and the omega-3 families of essential fatty acids. As mentioned previously, both families produce a series of prostaglandins that work in a complementary fashion and function well in this proportion.

The present North American ratio is much closer to 11 to 1, which means we are eating large amounts of linoleic acid (omega-6 family) and insufficient amounts of alpha-linolenic acid (omega-3 family). To attain the recommended 6 to 1 ratio, we can maintain a good intake of foods rich in linoleic acid (most nuts, seeds and their oils, whole grains) some of which are already common in our diet, but we should make sure to include more foods rich in alpha-linolenic acid and omega-3 fatty acids (fish and seafood, walnuts, soy, canola and linseed [flaxseed] oils, dark green leafy vegetables).

A daily diet made up of many different fresh, barely processed foods is the secret to quality, because essential fatty acids are very vulnerable to different industrial processes. The improved diet can include many servings of whole grains, fruit, and vegetables, some low-fat dairy products, beans, and fish. Without a drop of oil or any visible fat, such foods can satisfy all your basic needs for essential fatty acids (see the model menu Table 10). But you don't always need to be that strict. You can add other nutritious foods like nuts, seeds, and oils, but remember that essential fatty acids are found mainly in plant foods and are quite limited in foods of animal origin.

For example:

- 15 milliliters (1 tbsp) of butter contain 0.45 gram of essential fatty acids, while 15 milliliters (1 tbsp) of walnut oil contain 8.6 grams.
- 250 milliliters (1 cup) of ice cream supply 23 grams of total fat but only 1 gram of essential fatty acids.
- A portion of Quiche Lorraine (containing cream, eggs, ham), which supplies a total of 41 grams of fat, contains only 2.9 grams of essential fatty acids.
- 250 milliliters (1 cup) of cooked soybeans supply a total of 15 grams of fat and contain 8.7 grams of essential fatty acids.
- A wedge of cheddar cheese supplies a total of 10 grams of fat but only 0.2 gram of essential fatty acids.
- 15 milliliters (1 tbsp) of sunflower seeds supply a total of 4.3 grams of fat and have 2.8 grams of essential fatty acids.

Whole grain cereal products, because they retain their bran and germ, supply more essential fatty acids than white bread and refined cereals:

- A bowl of Swiss müesli supplies 3.03 grams of essential fatty acids, compared with a bowl of Corn Flakes, which has only 0.78 gram.
- A slice of whole-wheat bread contains 0.4 gram of essential fatty acids, while white bread contains only 0.22 gram.

Fruit and vegetables contain only a minute quantity of fat, but they do supply essential fatty acids.

At the other extreme, **meat and dairy products** supply a small amount of essential fatty acids in spite of their more significant content of total fat and saturated fat:

- 200 grams (7 oz) of plain yogurt made from partially skimmed milk supply 3.5 grams total fat, of which 2 grams are saturated fat, and only 0.1 gram is essential fatty acids.
- One whole egg contains a total of 6 grams of fat, of which only 0.7 gram is essential fatty acids.
- 30 grams (1 oz) of Swiss cheese contain 8 grams of total fat, of which only 0.3 gram is essential fatty acids.
- 90 grams (3 oz) of grilled veal contain 9 grams of total fat, of which only 0.6 gram is essential fatty acids.

Fish and seafood contain another type of fat and are proportionally richer in essential fatty acids than meats are:

- 90 grams (3 oz) of salmon supply 5 grams of fat, of which 1.9 grams are essential fatty acids.
- 90 grams (3 oz) of crabmeat supply 3 grams of fat, of which 0.5 gram is essential fatty acids.

Unfortunately these two essential fatty acids react to heat, to the refining process, and to oxidation, and often lose the battle against other fats in the diet. When foods are hydrogenated and/or deep-fried, essential fatty acids are the losers; they partly become *trans*-fatty acids and cannot perform their normal activities at the cellular level. The more processed and heated a food is, the more it loses its essential fatty acids and the more it becomes a liability. We see people at our nutrition clinic who eat amazing quantities of fried foods, cookies, and margarine, and they have elevated LDL (bad cholesterol) levels and very dry skins. More and more researchers are linking the lack of essential fatty acids to this type of eating and to several current diseases.

Your greatest challenge is to modulate and to protect your intake of essential fatty acids. To achieve the recommended ratio between omega-6 and the omega-3 fatty acids, you probably need to *increase* your intake of foods rich in omega-3 fatty acids. To protect their effectiveness at the cellular level, you need to *decrease* your intake of saturated fats and *avoid* hydrogenated fats.

This very basic menu below is composed of easy-to-find, high-quality foods that can fill your needs for essential fatty acids in the desired ratio of 6 to 1 without a drop of added oil or any visible fat.

Table 10 A model menu without any visible fat				
GROUP	GOOD CHOICES	TOTAL FAT	FATTY ACIDS	
		(g)	linoleic	alphalinolenic
			omega-6	omega-3
Cereal	1 bowl of cereal	1.2	1.66	0.12
products	3 slices of whole-grain bread	1.8	0.79	0.06
	250 ml/1 cup of brown rice	1.8	0.60	0.03
Vegetables	1 baked potato	0.2	0.05	0.02
	1 portion of broccoli and cauliflower	0.3	0.03	0.11
	1 romaine lettuce salad	0.2	0.04	0.08
	1 glass of orange juice	0.2	0.03	0.01
	1 bowl of strawberries	0.3	0.08	0.06
	1 pear	0.1	0.03	–
Milk	1 large glass of 1% milk	2.5	0.06	0.03
products	1 bowl of 0.2% yogurt	1.0	0.01	–
Meats and	90 g/3 oz of salmon	7.4	0.16	0.09
other proteins	1 bowl of cooked soybeans	7.7	3.85	0.52
TOTAL		24.7	7.39	1.13

This menu includes 6 servings of whole grains or whole cereal products, 6 to 7 servings of fruit and vegetables, 3 servings of low-fat dairy products, 1 serving of fish, and half a serving of soybeans. It provides less than 1,500 calories, and the fat content represents 15 percent of total calories.

You can round out the menu with other *good fats* such as olive or canola oil in a salad dressing, almonds or walnuts for a snack. By doing so, you will add fat and calories, but the quality of the fat is maintained.

If you decide to do things differently and add french fries, crackers, and cookies to this basic menu, you will be adding loads of *bad fats* and will compromise the positive impact of the essential fatty acids.

Quality, your first priority!

Before you start calculating every gram of fat in your daily diet, we suggest that you consider the *quality* of fats first.

Good fats are the fats that work on cellular growth, development, and maintenance, provide definite health benefits, and trigger no harmful reactions in our bodies. After having evaluated the impact of different fats on cardiovascular disease, cancers, and the immune system, we developed a list of *good fats* that comprises foods rich in monounsaturated fats (olive oil, canola oil, hazelnut oil, almonds, avocados), foods rich in alpha-linolenic acid (linseed and canola oil, soya, walnuts, dark green leafy vegetables), and foods rich in other omega-3 fatty acids (fish, algae, and seafood).

Do not forget, however, that even with good fats, the fresher the food, the better. Industrial processing and high cooking temperatures always affect some of their attributes.

Bad fats are fats that have been processed to the extent that they have lost their original composition and behavior at the cellular level. They compete with the essential fatty acids by disturbing the body's natural way of processing fats. They have been shown to cause trouble in the arteries as well as in the immune system. Bad fats comprise all foods that contain hydrogenated fats and *trans*-fatty acids.

Some fats are neither good nor bad by our definition: they are naturally found in certain foods and are quite abundant in our present diet — they can cause problems when eaten in excess.

Foods rich in **saturated fats** (meat, poultry, eggs, dairy products, butter) are neither good nor bad. They have very little effect on cellular growth, development, and maintenance; they have been shown to increase the LDL (bad cholesterol) in vulnerable individuals; and they compete with essential fatty acids when eaten in large quantities. Naturally present in our food supply since the beginning of time, they can play a complementary role *when there is no blood cholesterol problem*. But if your cholesterol level is too high, avoid saturated fats as much as possible.

Foods rich in **polyunsaturated fatty acids of the omega-6 family** (most vegetable oils such as corn, sunflower, safflower) do promote cellular growth, development, and maintenance but do not always help our immune system. Their great vulnerability to oxidation, their promoting effect on tumor growth in animal species, and their negative impact on the HDL (good cholesterol) explain this intermediate classification. Having been the health professional's first choice for many years, they still play a vital role but should not overshadow the omega-3 family.

Tropical oils have been severely criticized in recent years. They are rich in saturated fatty acids, work very little at cellular growth, development, and maintenance. Palm oil, which contains interesting amounts of antioxidants, should not be lumped together with coconut oil or palm kernel oil. Its composition is quite different. When not hydrogenated, palm oil can be quite useful in certain developing countries. Other tropical oils have little role to play.

Planning for quality

If you are healthy and have no weight problem, give priority to the *good fats*, with a diet rich in whole grains, fruits and vegetables, beans and tofu, fish, and some lean meats, poultry, and low-fat dairy products. Do not worry too much about the quantity.

If you are healthy but have a weight problem, forget about counting calories (it never works). Budget your grams of *good fats* and lose weight the healthy way. Low-fat foods such as grains and breads, beans, fruits, and vegetables are unlimited! At our nutrition clinic, we maintain an antidiet philosophy but have been using this "budget good fats" approach for the past two years. Patients find this type of diet quite satisfying and many have lost weight.

If you suffer from a serious cardiovascular problem or cancer, choose only good fats, but limit the total quantity. Your diet should come close to the model in Table 10 and will contain very little visible fat.

If you enjoy eating fried foods, margarine, cookies, chips, and crackers every day, your load of *bad fats* is significant, and you are seriously handicapping the essential fatty acids at the cellular level.

---

*It is healthful to eat the **good fats**:*
- *Foods rich in monounsaturates (olive oil, canola oil, almonds, avocado).*
- *Foods rich in alpha-linolenic acid (linseed oil, soybeans, walnuts, dark green leafy vegetables).*
- *Other foods rich in the other omega-3 fatty acids (fish and seafood).*

*It is not advantageous to eat the **bad fats** in foods rich in hydrogenated fats.*

*It is wise to limit foods rich in **saturated fats** (meat, poultry, dairy products, and butter) because of their competitiveness with the essential fatty acids. At present, these fats are too abundant in our diet.*

*It is also wise to limit foods rich in **polyunsaturated fatty acids from the omega-6 family** (sunflower, safflower, corn oils) because of their competitiveness with the omega-3 family.*

6

Labels Don't Tell the Whole Story

Labels give us more information than ever, but they don't always tell the truth, and nothing but the truth! They say what the law allows them to say, and nothing more!

Manufacturers have listed ingredients for years, but now they can insert nutrition claims such as "low in fat," "without fat," "low in saturated fat," "cholesterol-free," "light." Such claims attract our attention but often leave us quite confused. What does "no cholesterol" really mean? Is it better to buy foods "low in fat" or "low in saturated fat"?

The good news is that these claims must respect specific government regulations issued by Health and Welfare Canada in 1991. The bad news is that Canadian labels are still under review to see if they conform to the Canada-U.S. Trade Agreement, while revamped U.S. labels appeared in May 1994. Nevertheless, the nutrition jargon is quite similar.

To help you understand this jargon, we will first zoom in on the general nutrition information charts that appear on packaging. Then we will review claims used in relation to fat and permitted by 1991 Canadian regulations.

The general nutrition chart

All packaging that provides a nutrition claim regarding fat, or any other claim, must have a general nutrition chart. The following chart provides information on the main nutritional elements found in one small muffin.

```
┌─────────────────────────────────────────────────┐
│           NUTRITIONAL INFORMATION:              │
│          PER 50 g SERVING  (1 MUFFIN)           │
├─────────────────────────────────────────────────┤
│  ENERGY ...............................120 cal/500 kJ │
│  PROTEIN................................................2.2g │
│  FAT ......................................................1.5g │
│      POLYUNSATURATES .........................0.6g │
│      MONOUNSATURATES ........................0.5g │
│      SATURATES........................................0.2g │
│      CHOLESTEROL .................................0mg │
│  CARBOHYDRATES.................................26g │
│      DIETARY FIBER...............................2.0g │
└─────────────────────────────────────────────────┘
```

1. The values given on the chart always describe the contents for **one serving**: one muffin, one slice of bread, twenty french fries.

2. Energy, the first element on the chart, is expressed in **calories** (cal) or in kilojoules (kJ). The term *calorie* is an imperial-system measurement (just like cup, ounce, pound) while the term kilojoules is a metric measurement (just like milliliters, grams, kilograms). To convert from imperial to metric, multiply the calories by 4.18.

3. The content in **protein, fat**, and **carbohydrates** for one serving is expressed in **grams**. These three nutritional elements supply the calories in our foods.

4. When a statement or claim concerning the **fat** appears on the packaging, the label must also give a detailed description of the different fats present in the food. The amount of **saturated, monounsaturated**, and **polyunsaturated** fats, as well as the amount of cholesterol, are listed in the chart.

The total fatty acids does not always correspond to the total fat content because of the absence of information on *trans*-fatty acids that are in the food but never appear on the label. We consider that such information would be most useful for the health of Canadians and have asked Health and Welfare Canada to consider adding this crucial information to labels.

"lower in fat"

"Lower in fat" and "low fat" mean the same thing according to the law. When you see "low fat" on a label, it means that a serving does not supply more than 3 grams of fat per serving.

We examined the label of a bran-muffin mix that carried such a claim and concluded that the law was respected in this case, since one small muffin prepared with the mix supplied 1.5 grams of fat (the law allows up to 3 grams).

NUTRITIONAL INFORMATION: PER 50 g SERVING (1 MUFFIN)	
ENERGY	120 cal/500 kJ
PROTEIN	2.2g
FAT	1.5g
POLYUNSATURATES	0.6g
MONOUNSATURATES	0.5g
SATURATES	0.2g
CHOLESTEROL	0mg
CARBOHYDRATES	26g
DIETARY FIBER	2.0g

The food industry uses two methods of reducing fat in a food product. The first eliminates *part of* or *all* the fat present in a food: partially skimmed or totally skimmed milk, for example. The second method consists of withdrawing fat and replacing it with multiple additives (indicated by italics in the lists of ingredients on the following pages). The low-fat muffin mix is an illustration of the second method. Look at the list of ingredients:

List of ingredients: wheat flour, sugar, brown sugar, oat bran, wheat bran, soya, cotyledon fiber, vegetable oil, dextrose, baking powder, dried molasses preparation (blackstrap molasses, soya flour, wheat starch, soybean oil, *silicon dioxide*, hydroxylated lecithin), salt, rice bran, corn bran, oat flour, lecithin, skim milk powder, color, modified starch, spices, *polyglycerol esters of fatty acids, guar gum, artificial flavor*.

If you compare this "low-fat" muffin made from the mix to a small homemade muffin, you would find that the mix contains 3.4 grams less fat. But is this savings nutritionally valid? Not if we prepared a homemade muffin with a *good* fat such as canola oil.

Table 11 presents other foods labeled low in fat found on the market.

Table 11 Some foods labeled "low fat"	
FOODS	BRANDS
Breakfast cereals	All Bran, Cruncheroos, Froot Loops, Frosted Flakes, Fruit Full Bran, Just Right, Mini Wheats, Raisin Bran, Rice Krispies, Special K, Honey Nuts, Apple and Cinnamon Wheats, Balance Multibran, 100% Bran, Raisin Wheats, Shreddies, Fibre First, Corn Pops, Fruit Marshmallow, Trix, Crispix, Common Sense, Harvest Crunch, Hillsborough Mills
Muffin Mix	Robin Hood, Quaker
Breads and crackers	Weight Watchers, Premium plus, McCormicks, Millwheat

Whether they carry this claim or not, breakfast cereals, bread, and rice never contain much fat. For the time being, this particular claim seems of little use.

"fat free"

A "fat free" food contains less than one-tenth of a gram of fat per 100 grams.

A fat-free Italian salad dressing contains no trace of fat compared to a regular salad dressing, which contains 5 grams. But let's look at the list of ingredients and the nutritional analysis.

NUTRITIONAL INFORMATION: 15 ml SERVING (1 tbsp)
ENERGY ....4 cal/16 kJ
PROTEIN...0.1g
FAT 0g
POLYUNSATURATES 0g
MONOUNSATURATES 0g
SATURATES...0g
CHOLESTEROL 0mg
CARBOHYDRATE 0.7g

List of ingredients: water, white vinegar, lemon juice, *microcrystalline cellulose*, salt, dehydrated garlic, dehydrated onion, spices, natural flavor enhancer, *xanthan gum, cellulose gum*.

This dressing has no fat but contains more water, concentrated lemon juice, and a wide range of additives to replace the canola or soya oil present in a regular salad dressing. The claim is accurate, but is it really an advantage to replace all the oil with food additives? Are we swapping quantity of fat for a loss of nutritional quality?

There are so many ways to enhance the flavor of a salad. Balsamic vinegar does wonders for fresh tomato slices; a classic dressing made with an extra-virgin olive oil is delicious on crisp greens.

Table 12 lists foods labeled "fat free" on the market.

Table 12 Some foods labeled "fat free"	
FOODS	BRANDS
Desserts	Sealtest Sherbet
Salad dressing	Excelle, Chelton House
Yogurt	Sealtest, Silhouette, Astro

"low in saturated fats"

When you see a food labeled "low in saturated fats," it means that this food should provide in one serving:

- No more than 2 grams of saturated fatty acids.
- No more than 15 percent of calories from saturated fats.

One — a popular brand of french fries labeled "low in saturated fats," — contained the following ingredients:

List of ingredients: potatoes, *partially hydrogenated* canola and/or soybean oil, *dextrose, sodium acid pyrophosphate.*

NUTRITION INFORMATION: PER 100 g SERVING	
ENERGY	155 cal/650 kJ
PROTEIN	2.3g
FAT	4.5g
POLYUNSATURATES	0.3g
MONOUNSATURATES	2.3g
SATURATES	1.0g
CHOLESTEROL	0mg
CARBOHYDRATE	26g
SODIUM	47mg
POTASSIUM	319mg

A single serving of these fries gives you 1 gram of *saturated* fat, which supplies 6 percent of total calories. A serving of regular frozen french fries would give more than 4 grams of saturated fat, which supply 17 percent of calories.

Although they are "low in saturated fats," these fries still contain 5 grams of total fat per serving, while a raw potato contains one-tenth of a gram, which is fifty times less.

Until quite recently, french fries were prepared by cooking potatoes in boiling lard, an animal fat rich in saturated fatty acids. To lessen the saturated fat in the new fries, the industry now uses partially hydrogenated vegetable oil. It resolves one problem but causes another, since the use of hydrogenated fat brings with it the formation of *trans*-fatty acids.

Table 13 Some foods labeled "low in saturated fat"	
FOODS	BRANDS
Crackers	Christie's Premium Plus, Crispers, Croque en blé, Fins au blé, Ritz crackers, Bitelife's Snacking Crackers, Wheat Bubbles
Snack foods	Pringles, Bavarian Rold Gold Pretzels
French fries	McCain
Oil	Becel
Margarine	Imperial, Parkay Gold, Blue Bonnet, Fleischmann's
Cake mix	Duncan Hines
Salad dressings	Kraft, Hidden Valley

We found that foods "low in saturated fats" were not necessarily "low in fat"; quite the contrary! Foods such as chips, fries, oil, margarine, salad dressings all carry the claim "low in saturated fats." Many of these foods were prepared with hydrogenated fat. In fact, these foods provide less saturated fats but more hydrogenated fats . . . and more *trans*-fatty acids. Where is the health benefit?

"cholesterol free"

"Cholesterol free" foods don't necessarily provide a solution for people who wish to lower their blood cholesterol levels. Such foods contain:

- No more than 3 mg of cholesterol per 100 g.
- Not more than 2 grams per serving, or 15 percent of calories, coming from saturated fatty acids.

One salad dressing that had a "cholesterol free" label contained no cholesterol and very little saturated fatty acids.

NUTRITION INFORMATION: PER 15 ml (1 tbsp) SERVING
ENERGY ....36 cal/150 kJ
PROTEIN...0g
FAT 3.1g
POLYUNSATURATES 1.0g
MONOUNSATURATES 1.7g
SATURATES...................................0.2g
CHOLESTEROL...0mg
CARBOHYDRATES...................................2.4g

List of ingredients: water, canola oil, sugar, white vinegar, modified corn starch, salt, *microcrystalline cellulose*, mustard flour, egg white, color, *sodium carboxymethyl cellulose*, sodium caseinate, *xanthan gum*, spices, calcium disodium EDTA.

To eliminate the cholesterol from this dressing, the food industry replaced egg yolks rich in cholesterol with egg whites, which are always fat free, and substituted a few additives (in *italic* in the list of ingredients). This substitution saves 3 grams of fat per serving.

Never forget that this claim is often found on foods that are rich in fat and never had any trace of cholesterol. How confusing!

Before consuming any food claiming to be "cholesterol free," remember that cholesterol is found exclusively in foods of animal origin. No vegetable oil, whatever the source, ever contains any.

Table 14 Some foods labeled "cholesterol free"	
FOODS	BRANDS
Crackers	Melba toasts and sticks, Christies Croque en blé and Fins au blé, Wheatsworth, Mulino Bianco, Rusks, BiteLife
Breakfast cereals	Apple & Cinnamon Wheats, Shredded Wheat 'n Bran, Millwheat
Oils	Crisco, Primo, Unico, Bertolli, Becel, Montini Brand, Liberty, La Perla
Margarines	Country Crock, Nico
Cake and muffin mix	Duncan Hines, Betty Crocker
Breads	Weight Watchers, Dempster's, Hollywood, Wonder, Country Harvest
Puddings	Magic Moment
Salad dressings	Miracle Whip, Village
Other	Pam

"light" or "lightened"

The claims "light" or "lightened" have many different meanings. They can describe different characteristics in one food such as:

1. Physical aspects

- Light in color: Light brown rum
- Light in texture: Light High Liner supper
- Light in flavor: Bertolli Extra Light olive oil

The label has to clearly identify what aspect of the food is light or lighter; in reality, the information is there but in very small print.

In the case of extra-light olive oil the claim has baffled many consumers, who honestly believe they have found a low-cal oil! This cleverly marketed oil contains just as many calories and fat as the regular one; only the flavor is lighter as a result of significant refining.

PURE OLIVE OIL EXTRA LIGHT TASTE
Just a whisper of flavor, ideal for today's lighter dishes
NUTRITION INFORMATION:
PER 14 ml (1 tbsp) SERVING

FAT 12.8g
    POLYUNSATURATES 1.2g
    MONOUNSATURATES 9.8g
    SATURATES..1.8g
    CHOLESTEROL...0mg
SODIUM 0mg
POTASSIUM...0mg

2. Nutritional characteristics

- Lower in calories: Jell-O Light
- Lower in salt content: Lipton concentrated bouillon
- Lower in sugar content: Vachon's light fruit garnish
- Lower in fat content: Beatrice light yogurt, 0.5 percent less fat.

The use of the term "light" must then respond to very specific standards. With regard to fats, the claim "light" can only be used to describe two different types of foods:

- A food with low fat content. Remember the muffin that was "low in fat," because it contained less than 3 grams of fat per portion? The claims "light" or "low" fat mean the same thing, in this case.
- A food whose fat content has been reduced by at least 25 percent when compared with the regular food. Cheez Whiz *Light* claims that it contains *30 percent less fat* than the regular product; in effect, it does contain 2.4 grams less fat than the regular product and deserves the claim "light."

NUTRITION INFORMATION: per 30 ml (2 tbsp) SERVING
ENERGY ....77 cal/320 kJ
PROTEIN 5.5g
FAT 4.8g
CARBOHYDRATE 3.0g

The term "light" has so many different meanings that it is a confusing claim even to nutritionists.

Table 15 Some foods labeled "light"	
FOODS	BRANDS
Crackers	Wasa
Delicatessen	Maple Leaf, La Belle Fermière, Lifestyle Schneiders
Snacks	Pringles
Jam	Double-fruits, Habitant
Cheese	Kraft Philadelphia
Fruit garnish	E.D. Smith
Popcorn	Pop-secret Betty Crocker, Orville Redenbachers, Act II Lite
Mayonnaise	Hellmann's, Kraft
Margarine	Safflo

"pure," "100% pure," "100%"

Amazingly, these three claims can also mean many different things:

- That the food is not contaminated or an imitation and that it contains only the substances or ingredients expected. Corn oil that is "100% pure" contains only oil from corn and cannot contain any preservative or color. Pure vegetable oil, whether it is composed of one vegetable oil or a mixture of unidentified vegetable oils, cannot contain any other ingredient.
- That one of the ingredients in the product is 100 percent pure.

The claim "made from 100 % soya oil" found on some margarines does not mean that the margarine is made uniquely with soybean oil. In fact, one brand contains 80 percent soya oil, both liquid and hydrogenated, buttermilk, and whey (nonfat solids 1.4 percent), salt, vegetable monoglycerides, and soybean lecithin, potassium sorbate, lactic cultures, beta-carotene, BHA and BHT, Vitamin A palmitate, and vitamin D$_3$.

Nutrition claims may respect the law, but they do not necessarily tell the whole truth. We have found that they don't really help us detect good and bad fats. Luckily, we can turn to the list of ingredients.

7

Fats on the Market

Every time you buy foods at the grocery store or make food choices in restaurants and at home, you wonder if you are eating the right fats. Even after reading the first six chapters of this book, you may still be wondering what fats to choose or not to choose from now on.

This chapter summarizes technical details on the different oils, butters, and margarines. It also presents the results of our unique series of analyses done on cold-pressed oils.

Under each product you'll find the composition in fatty acids, the nutritional value, the impact on blood cholesterol, as well as other effects; brief tips on the culinary uses and storage of these fats are also included. Chapter 9 provides more information on what foods to buy, how to plan menus, and how to cook the healthier way.

Butter

Butter has been part of the human diet for a very long time. It has a secure place in various cuisines and still reigns over French cuisine (see "The French paradox" in chapter 5).

Production

You can prepare butter in your own kitchen with very cold fresh cream; you beat it until the molecules start to cluster and the cream becomes a thick, compact mass. You then discard the liquid part, the buttermilk, and save the solid part, the butter. Industrial production is essentially the same process.

Composition:	
Saturates	51%
Polyunsaturates	3%
Monounsaturates	24%

Nutritional value for 10 g (2 tsp):
> 72 calories
> 8.1 g fat
> 0.3 g polyunsaturates
> 2.4 g monounsaturates
> 5 g saturates
> 22 mg of cholesterol
> 0 mg vitamin E

Effect on blood cholesterol: Butter, rich in saturated fatty acids, raises total blood cholesterol and LDL (bad cholesterol) in vulnerable individuals.

Other impact: Even if you don't have high blood cholesterol, butter remains a rich source of saturated fat that is neither a *good* fat nor a *bad* fat. A moderate intake is acceptable but not a must.

Culinary tips

It is always best to have butter raw, not cooked. Use it sparingly on cooked foods instead of frying food in it. High cooking temperatures are never recommended; when cooked butter turns brown, you are in trouble!

Storage tips
- Keep refrigerated.
- Discard if rancid.

Different butters

Light butter ("pure and wholesome" type) contains 39 percent fat, which represents a 50 percent reduction in fat and calories compared with regular butter; the list of ingredients comprises butter, dairy substances, water, salt, distilled monoglycerides, carob gum, potassium sorbate, citric acid, and coloring.

Half-salted butter contains 50 percent less salt than regular butter.

Unsalted or *sweet* butter contains no added salt.

Cultured butter is an unsalted butter with bacterial culture added before churning.

Seasoned butter is regular butter laced with seasonings such as herbs or spices.

Whipped butter is regular butter that has been churned in such a way as to let air penetrate, which has the effect of increasing its volume and rendering it softer and creamier.

Margarines

Believe it or not, margarine was developed during a competition launched by Napoleon III in order to find "a fitting product to replace butter," as there was not enough butter to meet public demand. Although commercial production of margarine started at the end of the nineteenth century, the French did not really adopt this product until quite recently (see "The French paradox" in chapter 5).

Production

The majority of margarines are made from liquid vegetable oils that are first refined and then chemically processed to become a semi-solid stable fat. These margarines, stick margarines more than tub margarines, contain a fair amount of hydrogenated fat and *trans*-fatty acids.

Preservatives, antioxidants, additives, natural and artificial flavorings, and coloring are added.

Composition	
The fatty acid content varies depending on the oils used.	
Soft margarines may contain:	
Polyunsaturates	10 to 35%
Monounsaturates	28 to 40%
Saturates	10 to 12%
Trans-fatty acids	1 to 20%
Hard margarines may contain:	
Polyunsaturates	3 to 21%
Monounsaturates	34 to 42%
Saturates	12 to 16%
Trans-fatty acids	1 to 30%

Nutritional value for 10 g (2 tsp):
(the nutritional value corresponds to a margarine prepared with soybean oil)

　　72 calories
　　8 g fat
　　3.2 g polyunsaturates

2.2 g monounsaturates
1.4 g saturates
1.2 g *trans*-fatty acids
no trace of cholesterol
0.7 mg vitamin E (alpha-tocopherol)

Effect on blood cholesterol: Recent research shows that *trans*-fatty acids, present in most margarines, raise LDL (bad cholesterol) and lower HDL (good cholesterol).

Studies by Dr. Walter Willett, made over eight years with more than 80,000 nurses (see chapter 2), indicate that 20 g (4 tsp) of hydrogenated margarine per day increases the risk of heart disease by 60 percent.

Other impact: Because of their *trans*-fatty acids, hydrogenated margarines are considered a source of *bad* fats; such fats compete with essential fatty acids and affect cellular interactions (see chapter 4). They do not belong in a healthy diet.

Storage tips
• Keep refrigerated.

Canadian regulations
The Food and Drugs Act does not require manufacturers to declare the presence of *trans*-fatty acids in their margarine.

Hard (stick) or soft (tub) margarines
These two types of margarines contain the same amount of calories and the same amount of fat. The main difference is in their consistency and their degree of hydrogenation, a hard margarine containing approximately twice the amount of hydrogenated fat.

So, the harder a margarine is, the more hydrogenated it is, the more *trans*-fatty acids it contains, and the more it competes with the essential fatty acids.

Nonhydrogenated margarines
Certain margarines are made *without hydrogenation*. These margarines, made with one oil or mixtures of refined oils, have a higher

content of saturated refined palm oil than most margarines. Part of the palm oil is fractionated, crystallized, and mixed with the other oils. To obtain a more uniform texture, the oils are then *transesterified*. This is a physical modification that rearranges the different fatty acids on the fat molecule but does not seem to affect their attributes. Brand names for such margarines include Becel, Olivina, Nuvel.

In our view, these new margarines do not represent a healthy choice because they are fabricated with refined and highly processed oils and because their long-term health impact is still a question mark.

Low-calorie margarines

Some margarines, called "light" or "lo-cal," *contain half the oil* and much more water than regular margarines. They provide half the fat and half the calories.

Low-sodium margarines

These margarines contain as many calories and fat as regular margarine but contain 200 times less salt. Some so-called "semi-soft" margarines contain two to three times less salt than a regular margarine, but just as much fat.

Refined Oils

Refined oils, the ones usually available at the grocery store, can be compared to *white* flour, which has undergone modifications that cause various nutritional losses.

Production

Makers of refined oils use seeds grown the traditional way using fertilizers and pesticides. After they are hulled, they are heated to between 80° and 120°C (176° and 248°F) to allow maximal extraction of the oil; this extraction is made under pressure and with the help of a solvent.

At this stage, the extracted oil is crude and unsuitable for human consumption. The crude oil still contains some solvent and some undesirable substances that can easily become rancid. It then undergoes a number of physical and chemical treatments: degumming by heating the oil to between 60° and 90°C (140° and 194°F) to remove substances such as lecithin, natural oxidants, and minerals; refining by heating the oil to 75°C (167°F) to eliminate free fatty acids; bleaching by heating the oil to between 80° and 100°C (176° and 212°F) to eliminate any trace of pigments; deodorizing by heating the oil to between 240° and 270°C (464° and 518°F) to subtract any leftover odor or taste. These modifications made at high temperatures cause the formation of *trans*-fatty acids. Once the oil has lost most of its original color, taste, and odor, it is bottled and sealed.

Effects of refining

Vitamin E, lecithin, sterols, phenols, and several pigments, among other components, are negatively affected by the whole refining process. Analyses of crude oil extracts (oils that have been extracted from plants but have not gone through the refining process) have shown a greater resistance to auto-oxidation due to the presence of active, naturally occurring antioxidants. These active antioxidants and other substances constitute the *little things that make a difference* in the total value of an oil; they are negatively affected by the rest of the refining process. High temperatures during the refining process are also responsible for the formation of undesirable *trans*-fatty acids, especially in oils rich in alpha-linolenic acid such as soybean or canola oils. The story is still incomplete but research goes on.

Cold-pressed Oils

Cold-pressed oils, labeled as such and usually sold in health-food stores, are comparable to stone-ground whole wheat flour, which has undergone very little processing and very little nutritive losses.

Cold-pressed oils have been talked about for many years, but they have not been the subject of much research except for extra-virgin olive oil. We have been quite interested in this topic since 1986. We were getting many requests for information and were very curious, so we conducted two series of analyses, in 1989 and in 1992. For these analyses, we chose sunflower oil because of its great availability.

Cold pressing is an ancient traditional method in which the seeds are not heated before, during, or after the pressing process. Seeds are selected, cleaned, and crushed; they are then mechanically pressed at a slow pace to limit friction and avoid elevating temperatures above 60°C. The oil then rests for approximately twenty-four hours before it is filtered and bottled. Its color, taste, and odor are much more pronounced than those of refined oils. In North America, no regulations apply to such a procedure. Switzerland is one of the only countries that has strict regulations.

In 1989, we conducted a very simple test; we bought four bottles of sunflower oil labeled *cold-pressed* at a health-food store and one bottle of refined oil at the supermarket. We transferred all the oils to coded bottles and used two separate laboratories to analyze the samples. The results showed that of the four labeled cold-pressed, two were not; they contained no free fatty acids, which meant that they had been refined. The real cold-pressed oils had much higher levels of vitamin E. Even though no Canadian regulations exist to protect the consumer against such fraud, real cold-pressed oils still seem more advantageous.

To answer more of our questions, a second series of tests was done in 1992 in collaboration with the department of nutrition at the University of Montreal. Sunflower seeds were obtained from Canamara Foods in Saskatchewan as was a liter of freshly refined oil. We brought the sunflower seeds to Quebec City to have them mechanically pressed at Orphé's, one of the few Canadian companies that produces and sells cold-pressed oils. We then bought commercial sunflower oils — four bottles labeled cold-pressed and four regular bottles — transferred the eleven different oils to seven series of coded bottles and distributed all samples to the different research centers within ten days. Dr. Mohsen Meydani at Tufts in Boston analyzed the oils for their vitamin E content. Dr. Victor Gavino at the University of Montreal and Dr. Stan Kubow at McGill University measured the content of *trans*-fatty acids using two different methods in their respective labs. Dr. Kubow also analyzed the beta-sitosterol content (an interesting substance that blocks cholesterol absorption). Novalab, a commercial laboratory, looked at some pesticides and hexane residues.

The results established significant differences between the two types of oils:

- Cold-pressed oils contained 50 percent more alpha-tocopherol and 25 percent more gamma-tocopherol (two different forms of vitamin E) than refined oils; this additional amount of antioxidants is quite significant and can provide better protection against oxidation, a very critical problem with polyunsaturates.
- Cold-pressed oils contained 45 percent more beta-sitosterols than refined oils; beta-sitosterols are substances, naturally found in plants, that have been shown to inhibit cholesterol absorption. They are so effective that in the seventies, beta-sitosterols were used as the active ingredient in several medications to reduce cholesterol.
- Even though the amounts are minute in both types of oil, refined oils contained 4 1/2 times more *trans*-fatty acids than the cold-pressed oils.

Another series of analyses done in France by Robert Wolff on eight salad dressings and five food samples made with soybean or rapeseed oils has shown that with only one exception, all refined oils contained a significant amount of *trans*-fatty acids. *Trans*-fatty acids are definitely *bad* fats, and the less we eat, the better.

- No hexane residues were found in any of our samples.
- No carbamate residues (carbaryl and carbofuran) were detected in the any of our samples. (We had identified two specific pesticides for analyses because we could not afford to analyze the sixty different substances in the carbamate family.)

Nutritional impact

Our results provide evidence that there is a nutritional benefit to choosing a cold-pressed oil because of a much higher antioxidant content (vitamin E), a higher beta-sitosterol content, which inhibits the absorption of cholesterol, and a significantly lower content of *trans*-fatty acids.

Our analyses did not look into all the other potentially interesting ingredients present in oils, but they confirm the superior qualities of truly cold-pressed oils. Despite these definite benefits, no regulation protects the Canadian consumer against oils falsely labeled "cold-pressed."

CANOLA OIL

Availability

Canola oil, a relative newcomer on the oil scene, is produced from genetically altered rapeseed, a plant that grows in the Prairies. It is used in many oil mixtures, margarines, and other food products. You can find refined canola oil quite easily in grocery stores, and cold-pressed canola oil in health-food stores.

Composition	
Polyunsaturates	36% (26% omega-6, 10% omega-3)
Monounsaturates	58%
Saturates	6%

Nutritional value for 10 ml (2 tsp):
(value given for refined canola)
83 calories
9.2 g fat
0.6 g saturates
5.8 g monounsaturates
2.8 g polyunsaturates
no trace of cholesterol
1.9 mg vitamin E (alpha-tocopherol)

Effects on blood cholesterol: Lowers LDL (bad cholesterol) and protects HDL (good cholesterol).

Other impact: Canola oil is considered a good fat because of its rich content in monounsaturated and omega-3 fatty acids. It is even more healthful when cold-pressed.

Culinary tips

Use in salad dressings or in marinades.
In cooking, it can tolerate some direct heat; can be used to lightly brown poultry, vegetables, fish and seafoods.
Can be used in baking muffins, cakes, breads.
Can be mixed with butter to make a healthful spread on toast.

Storage tips
- Buy in small quantities.
- Protect from light and keep in a dark place.
- Protect from air and close bottle after use.
- Keep in a cool place; keep in refrigerator if cold-pressed.
- Check the expiry date if there is one.

CORN OIL

Availability

You can find refined corn oil very easily in grocery stores and, very seldom, cold-pressed corn oil in health-food stores.

Composition	
Polyunsaturates	62% (61% omega-6 , 1% omega-3)
Monounsaturates	25%
Saturates	13%

Nutritional value for 10 ml (2 tsp):
(values are given for refined oil)
>   80 calories
>   9.1 g fat
>   1.1 g saturates
>   2.2 g monounsaturates
>   8.0 g polyunsaturates
>   no trace of cholesterol
>   1.3 mg vitamin E

Effects on blood cholesterol: Lowers total cholesterol, including HDL (good cholesterol).

Other impact: Because of its high content of omega-6 fatty acids, corn oil is neither a *good* nor a *bad* fat; a moderate intake is acceptable if so desired.

Culinary tips
Use in salad dressings.
Does not withstand cooking on direct heat.
Can be used in baking if desired.

Storage tips
- Buy in small quantities.
- Protect from light and keep in a cool dark place.
- Protect from air and close bottle immediately after use.
- Keep in the refrigerator if the oil is cold-pressed.
- Check the expiry date.

HAZELNUT OIL

Availability

Regular grocery stores do not sell this oil. You may find refined hazelnut oil in specialty shops and cold-pressed oil in health-food shops.

Composition	
Polyunsaturates	11% (omega-6)
Monounsaturates	79%
Saturates	7%

Nutritional value for 10 ml (2 tsp):
(values are given for refined oil)

> 80 calories
> 9.1 g fat
> 0.7 g saturates
> 7.1 g monounsaturates
> 0.9 g polyunsaturates
> no trace of cholesterol
> 4.7 mg vitamin E (alpha-tocopherol)

Effects on blood cholesterol: Lowers LDL (bad cholesterol) and protects HDL (good cholesterol).

Other impact: Because of its high content of monounsaturated fatty acid, hazelnut oil is considered a *good* fat.

Culinary tips

Use in salad dressings for fine-tasting salads.

Can be mixed with butter, half and half, for a healthful and tasty spread on toast!

Cook on low direct heat, if needed.

Can be used in baking pancakes, muffins, cakes.

Has a characteristic very fine taste.

Storage tips
- Buy in small quantities.
- Protect from light and keep in a dark place.
- Protect from air and close bottle after use.
- Keep in a cool place if cold-pressed.
- Check the expiry date.

Comment
Hazelnut oil is quite expensive.

LINSEED (FLAXSEED) OIL

Availabilty

Linseed oil is generally not found in grocery stores. You can find this oil in health-food stores in cold-pressed form.

Composition	
Polyunsaturates	68% (14% omega-6, 54% omega-3)
Monounsaturates	21%
Saturates	9%

Nutritional value for 10 ml (2 tsp):
(values are given for refined oil)

> 80 calories
> 9.1 g fat
> 0.9 g saturates
> 1.8 g monounsaturates
> 6.0 g polyunsaturates
> no trace of cholesterol
> vitamin E level unknown

Effects on blood cholesterol: Few studies have been carried out on this oil.

Other impact: Linseed oil, with its high omega-3 content, is distinct from all other oils. It seems to have a positive impact on the immune system. It is considered a *good* fat, but there is no benefit in consuming large quantities.

Culinary tips

Can be used in salad dressings, mixed with another oil, if desired.
Can be mixed with low-fat cheese and served as a spread.
Not at all appropriate for direct-heat cooking.
It is not advised for use in baked foods.
Has a distinct flavor.

Storage tips
- Buy in very small quantities — not more than 250 ml (8 fl oz).
- Protect from light and keep in a dark bottle.
- Protect from air and close bottle after use.
- Keep in refrigerator for a maximum of two months after purchase.
- Check the expiry date.

Comment
Linseed oil is expensive and spoils rapidly.

OLIVE OIL
Availability

You can easily find several types of olive oil on the market. Most of them are produced in Mediterranean countries that belong to the International Olive Oil Council, a trade organization that regulates the production and the labeling of olive oil. The different qualities of olive oil correspond to different degrees of acidity; the less acidity, the higher the quality.

- *Extra-virgin olive oil* corresponds to a *first cold-pressing* which is the highest quality. It contains very little acidity and has the finest and most pleasing taste.
- *Virgin olive oil* is also a cold-pressed olive oil that has not undergone any heat treatment. The level of acidity is very low.
- *Pure olive oil* contains more acidity. It is a mixture of refined olive oil that has been heated and 5 to 10 percent virgin olive oil.
- *Light olive oil* contains refined oil that has been heated. The taste is light and the quality is low.

Several brands, including Pastene, Bertolli, and Fillippo Berio, offer the whole range of olive oils, from pure to extra-virgin. Hence the importance of reading labels carefully.

Canada has no specific regulations or inspection protocol concerning such label claims.

Composition	
Polyunsaturates	9% (8% omega-6, 1% omega-3)
Monounsaturates	76%
Saturates	15%

Nutritional value for 10 ml (2 tsp):

> 80 calories
> 9.0 g fat
> 1.2 g saturates
> 6.6 g monounsaturates
> 0.6 g polyunsaturates
> no trace of cholesterol
> 1.1 mg vitamin E (alpha-tocopherol)

Effects on blood cholesterol: Lowers LDL (bad cholesterol), protects and sometimes increases HDL (good cholesterol).

Other impact: Because of its rich content in monounsaturated fatty acids and many other components when cold-pressed, extra-virgin olive oil is considered a *good* fat.

Culinary tips

Use in salads dressings and marinades.

Mix with lemon juice and sprinkle on cooked fish and seafood.

Mix with garlic and fresh basil to make pesto sauce.

Can be used for cooking on moderate heat; resistance to heat is even greater when oil is extra-virgin.

Can be used in baking.

Brush on pizza dough or on bread with a little garlic.

Storage tips

- Buy in small quantities.
- Protect from light and keep in a dark place.
- Protect from air and close bottle immediately after use.
- Keep in a cool place but not in the refrigerator.
- Check the expiry date.

PEANUT OIL

Availability

You can find refined peanut oil in grocery stores and cold-pressed peanut oil in health-food stores.

Composition	
Polyunsaturates	34% (omega-6)
Monounsaturates	48%
Saturates	18%

Nutritional value for 10 ml (2 tsp):
(values are given for refined oil)
>90 calories
>10 g fat
>1.9 g saturates
>4.5 g monounsaturates
>3.6 g polyunsaturates
>no trace of cholesterol
>1.1 mg vitamin E (alpha-tocopherol)

Effects on blood cholesterol: Few studies have been carried out on this oil.

Other impact: This oil is frequently referred to as the frying oil; its composition does not call for such usage. Individuals who are allergic to peanuts can react to peanut oil.

Culinary tips

Use in salad dressings and marinades.
Can be used to lightly brown or stir-fry poultry, fish, Chinese-style vegetables.
Can be used in baking muffins, cakes, pancakes, breads, cookies.
Has a characteristic flavor.

Storage tips

- Buy in small quantities.
- Protect from light and keep in a dark place.
- Protect from air and close bottle after use.
- Keep in a cool place.
- Check the expiry date.

SAFFLOWER OIL

Availability

You can find refined safflower oil in grocery stores and cold-pressed safflower oil in health-food stores.

Composition	
Polyunsaturates	78% (omega-6 and a trace of omega-3)
Monounsaturates	13%
Saturates	9%

Nutritional value for 10 ml (2 tsp):
(values are given for refined oil)
>   80 calories
>   9.0 g fat
>   0.8 g saturates
>   1.1 g monounsaturates
>   6.8 g polyunsaturates
>   no trace of cholesterol
>   3.4 mg vitamin E (alpha-tocopherol)

Effects on blood cholesterol: Lowers total cholesterol and HDL (good cholesterol).

Other impact: Because of its rich polyunsaturated content of omega-6, safflower is considered neither a *good* nor a *bad* fat. Can be used in small quantities, if desired.

Culinary tips

Use in salad dressings and some desserts because of its light taste.

It is not appropriate for cooking on direct heat.

Can be used in baking bread, cakes, muffins.

Has a very mild flavor.

Storage tips

- Buy in small quantities.
- Protect from light and keep in a dark bottle.
- Protect from air and close bottle after use.
- Keep in refrigerator if oil is cold-pressed; if not, keep in cool place.
- Check the expiry date.

SESAME OIL

Availability

You can find refined sesame oil in Chinese or Asian grocery stores, and cold-pressed sesame oil in health-food stores.

Composition	
Polyunsaturates	43% (omega-6 and traces of omega-3)
Monounsaturates	41%
Saturates	15%

Nutritional value for 10 ml (2 tsp):
(values are given for refined oil)
>   80 calories
>   9.1 g fat
>   1.3 g saturates
>   3.6 g monounsaturates
>   3.8 g polyunsaturates
>   no trace of cholesterol
>   0.15 mg vitamin E (alpha-tocopherol)

Effects on blood cholesterol: There is little information on this oil.

Other impact: A moderate intake can provide variety and flavor.

Culinary tips
Can be used in salad dressings.
Adds a characteristic flavor to bean sprouts and other salads.
Use sparingly in wok cooking for Asian dishes.
Can be used in baking.
Has a characteristic flavor.

Storage tips
>   • Buy in small quantities.
>   • Protect from light and keep in a dark place.
>   • Protect from air and close bottle after use.
>   • Keep in a cool place; keep in refrigerator if oil is cold-pressed.
>   • Check the expiry date.

SOYBEAN OIL

Availability

You can find refined soybean oil in grocery stores; often soybean oil is mixed with other oils and sold as vegetable oil.

Composition	
Polyunsaturates	58% (51% omega-6, 7% omega-3)
Monounsaturates	24%
Saturates	15%

Nutritional value for 10 ml (2 tsp):
(value given for refined soybean oil)
> 80 calories
> 9.1 g fat
> 1.3 g saturates
> 2.1 g monounsaturates
> 5.3 g polyunsaturates
> no trace of cholesterol
> 1.0 mg vitamin E (alpha tocopherol)

Effects on blood cholesterol: Lowers total cholesterol, including HDL (good cholesterol).

Other impact: In small quantities, can provide some omega-3 fatty acids.

Culinary tips

Can be used in salad dressings.
Does not withstand direct heat because of its high omega-6 and omega-3 content.
Can be used in baking muffins, pancakes.

Storage tips
> • Buy in small quantities.
> • Protect from light and keep in a dark place.
> • Protect from air and close bottle after use.
> • Keep in a cool place.
> • Check the expiry date.

SUNFLOWER OIL

Availability

You can find refined sunflower oil in grocery stores and cold-pressed sunflower oils in health-food stores.

Composition	
Polyunsaturates	69% (omega-6)
Monounsaturates	20%
Saturates	11%

Nutritional value for 10 ml (2 tsp):
(values are given for refined oil)

      83 calories
      9.2 g fat
      1.2 g saturates
      1.5 g monounsaturates
      6.5 g polyunsaturates
      no trace of cholesterol
      4.1 mg vitamin E (alpha-tocopherol)

Effects on blood cholesterol: Lowers total cholesterol, including HDL (good cholesterol).

Other impact: Can provide variety and flavor in small quantities.

Culinary tips

Use in salad dressings and marinades.
Does not tolerate direct heat at high temperatures.
Use in baking muffins, cakes, bread, cookies.
Has a very mild flavor.

Storage tips

• Buy in small quantities.
• Protect from light and keep in a dark place.
• Protect from air and close bottle immediately after use.
• Keep in the refrigerator if cold-pressed; if not, keep in a cool place.
• Check the expiry date.

WALNUT OIL

Availability

Walnut oil is not sold in regular grocery stores; you can find refined walnut oil in some gourmet shops or cold-pressed walnut oil in health-food stores. In France, used more frequently in salad dressings for divine salads!

Composition	
Polyunsaturates	66% (55% omega-6, 11% omega-3)
Monounsaturates	23%
Saturates	9%

Nutritional value for 10 ml (2 tsp):
(values given for refined oil)

     80 calories

     9.1 g fat

     0.8 g saturates

     2.1 g monounsaturates

     5.7 g polyunsaturates

     no trace of cholesterol

     0.07 mg vitamin E (alpha-tocopherol)

Effects on blood cholesterol: There is little information on this oil.

Culinary tips

Use in salad dressings.

Does not tolerate direct heat. It is inappropriate for cooking because of high omega-6 and omega-3 content.

Has a very unique flavor.

Storage tips

- Buy in small quantities.
- Protect from light and keep in a dark place.
- Protect from air and close bottle immediately after use.
- Keep in a cool place; keep in refrigerator if cold-pressed.
- Check the expiry date.

Comment

This oil is expensive.

TROPICAL OILS
(coconut, palm, palm kernel)

Availability

You cannot buy a bottle of tropical oil the way you can buy a bottle of olive oil, but the food industry uses tropical oils in significant amounts in many foods for taste, texture, and consistency at low cost. The tropical oil family includes palm oil, palm kernel oil, coconut oil, babassu oil. All these oils contain a fair amount of saturated fats but palm oil has distinct nutritional properties and cannot be lumped together with all the others.

Nutritional impact

Because of their high content in saturated fats, coconut and palm kernel oils increase total cholesterol, including LDL (bad cholesterol), and may lead to the formation of clots that block the arteries. Experts on palm oil such as Dr. Richard Cottrell of England disagree with the lumping together of all tropical oils and underline that none of the major experiments done until now have shown unequivocal adverse effects. We add that studies have been carried out with refined tropical oils.

Meanwhile, *unrefined* red palm oil is the richest known natural source of beta-carotene. It also contains important amounts of tocotrienol and tocopherol, two active antioxidants, and some beta-sitosterol, which can inhibit cholesterol absorption. When this oil is refined, the carotenes are lost almost completely; the other antioxidants are seriously reduced as well. In a country like India, the regular use of red palm oil could help eliminate the vitamin A deficiency, a wide-spread deficiency that leads to blindness at a very tender age.

In our country, the use of refined palm oil allows manufacturers to limit the hydrogenation process in many food products, which in turn decreases the amount of *trans*-fatty acids in some foods.

For these reasons, we do not consider palm oil in particular to be either a *bad* fat or a *good* fat.

Food products that contain them:
- Cookies of all sorts
- Shake 'n' Bake
- Some margarines
- Some cereals
- Some bakery products
- Some pizza-dough mixes

8

Supplements and Substitutes

Our body needs fat to function properly, and ideally, it gets it from foods rich in essential fatty acids of the omega-6 and omega-3 families. But as we discussed in the previous chapters, individuals may lack some of these fatty acids for several dietary and health reasons.

Luckily, some of these fats are sold in the form of supplements in drugstores and health-food stores. These existing fat supplements are classified into two categories: ones that supply fatty acids of the omega-6 family, and ones that supply fatty acids from the omega-3 family in the form of fish oils.

Evening primrose oil and borage seed oil are the best-known supplements for omega-6, cod liver oil and halibut liver oil for omega-3. (Fish oils now come in capsule form and are much easier to swallow than in the old days; they have very little aftertaste.)

Evening primrose oil and borage seed oil

Evening primrose oil is extracted from the flower that bears the same name, while borage seed oil is extracted from the seeds of borage. They both contain a very special fatty acid called gamma-linolenic acid. This oil is naturally present in human mother's milk, but it disappears from our diet after weaning; our body becomes capable of producing enough from linoleic acid, the omega-6 parent substance. But sometimes, the conversion from the parent derivative is seriously limited by too much saturated fat, too much hydrogenated fat, or too much alcohol in the diet, creating an insufficient supply of gamma-linolenic acid, a key element in the chain of omega-6 derivatives. Aging, intense periods of stress, or illnesses like diabetes or viral infections can also cause the same type of problem.

Numerous studies have looked at the impact of gamma-linolenic acid on the human body. They have shown that this very special fat enhances the production of some very useful prostaglandins, essential for female hormonal balance. It also protects the skin, the immune system, and cardiovascular system. Some researchers claim that a gamma-linolenic-acid deficiency can be detrimental to health in many ways; research is ongoing.

Evening primrose oil has been studied and used more extensively than borage seed oil. *CPS*, the compendium of pharmaceutical products, a working tool for health professionals that describes most medications sold in Canada, mentions that evening primrose oil can help relieve premenstrual tension symptoms. In our clinical practice we have recommended evening primrose oil to women with premenstrual problems along with vitamin B_6 and have seen good results. With individuals who had dry-skin problems, we have also had interesting results; within a month, we could see and feel the difference. Evening primrose oil can be useful in other skin problems, such as psoriasis, dermatitis, and eczema.

While we do not claim that evening primrose oil always works, there are no risks attached to a daily dose unless you suffer from epilepsy. It is harmless when ingested in the recommended amounts but can cause diarrhea when taken in large amounts. In any case it is best to take this supplement at mealtimes rather than on an empty stomach, to avoid possible nausea.

To do its work efficiently, gamma-linolenic acid needs zinc, pyridoxine (vitamin B_6), niacin (vitamin B_3) and vitamin C, which can be found in foods or supplements.

The market offers several evening primrose oil supplements; the quality can vary, so look for the following information on the label:

- A DIN code, which is the drug's identification number.
- A lot number.
- An expiry date.
- The precise composition.

Some evening primrose oil is sold in small quantities as cold-pressed oil. Verify if the oil comes from organically grown flowers. This does not guarantee quality, but it does denote a certain level of control.

According to a series of analyses carried out in France in 1992 by the inter-regional laboratory of Montpellier in connection with the prevention of fraud, some evening primrose oils did not even contain evening primrose oil, while others were from rancid and oxidized seeds. Only one brand met all the criteria of quality. The situation is perhaps different in Canada, but be sure to look for quality.

Borage seed oil contains an even larger amount of gamma-linolenic acid than evening primrose oil but is perhaps less efficient in enhancing the formation of useful prostaglandins. For the moment, there is little borage seed oil on the market.

Fish oils

In the first chapter, we saw that fish oils were used in research projects to treat certain illnesses. In general, researchers used fish-oil supplements that are not sold in Canada, and often, they used significant doses, but these researchers were competent and had the means to control their studies. It is not wise for you to increase your intake of fish oils without professional supervision; you can take too much and have side effects that can sometimes be worse than if you take too little.

Nevertheless, fish oils can be useful in reducing inflammation, slowing down the blood-clotting process, and stimulating the immune system. The best strategy to take advantage of these benefits is to increase your fish intake, fatty fish in particular: salmon, mackerel, sardines.

If you are allergic to or do not like this type of food, a fish-oil supplement can help you out. But even so, do not take just any oil.

In Canada, two fish oils have been approved and possess a DIN code. These are cod liver oil and halibut liver oil. Verify the expiry date on the label and lot number.

You can buy these supplements in capsule form. These oils also contain vitamins A and D, which are fat-soluble and can be toxic if taken in excessive quantities. As a measure of prudence, never exceed a dose of 400 IU of vitamin D per day, and during pregnancy, never take more than 10,000 IU of vitamin A per day.

One capsule of **cod liver oil** contains:

- omega-3 fatty acids
- 1,250 to 3,000 IU of vitamin A
- 100 to 300 IU vitamin D

One capsule of **halibut liver oil** contains:

- omega-3 fatty acids
- 5,000 to 10,000 IU of vitamin A
- 400 IU of vitamin D

Fat substitutes: the *new* fats

The food industry has once again overreacted to the fear of cholesterol and the diet obsession. It has created new fats that mimic the texture of real fat but no longer supply as many calories, nor as much fat.

In contrast to a simple additive, which is added to food in very small amounts, these new fats can potentially take up a very large place in tomorrow's diet.

While 57 percent of Americans believe in the appropriateness of such fat substitutes, we are less enthusiastic and still have many questions that need answers.

In Canada, only a few of the following fat substitutes are currently found in foods, while in the United States more of them are present: Dairy Light, Olestra, Salatrim, Simplesse; their names are listed as such in the list of ingredients.

Dairy Light

This fat substitute is esentially made from milk proteins that have been processed in such a way to replace cream and yet still provide a fat taste and texture. For the moment it is used in Parlour 1% Ice Cream. According to the company, which has patented the product, this new cream can be used in many other dairy and nondairy products.

Olestra

This product is composed of eight fatty acids attached to a molecule of sugar and is not absorbed by the body.

Olestra is used in the United States but is not yet accepted in Canada. Made by chemical synthesis, it has yet to be tested for safety. It can be used for chips and other fried foods. It provides no calories, no cholesterol, and no fat.

Salatrim

Salatrim is a new family of low-calorie fats made from a combination of short- and long-chain fatty acids. After interesterification of highly hydrogenated vegetable oils with triacylglycerols, a component of fatty acids, a new fat is formed with fewer calories (five instead of nine per gram). It can be liquid or solid, white or yellow, depending on the combination of fatty acids. It is not yet being used in food products but is suited for chocolate coatings for candy bars, sour cream, cheese, margarines, and spreads.

Simplesse™

This substitute is made from egg white and milk proteins that have been reduced to microparticles to simulate the texture of fat. It was ruled acceptable in Canada in February 1990 as a thickening agent and texture modifier for frozen desserts. No evidence was required to ensure the absence of undesirable effects on health.

Simplesse can be incorporated into sour cream, dips, ice cream, butter, yogurt, cheese, icing, refrigerated desserts, salad dressings, mayonnaise, and margarine.

However, Simplesse cannot be used for frying.

Other substances such as *gums*, *soluble fibers*, and *starches* are used to thicken ice creams and several food products. Although these products have been accepted for a long time as food additives or ingredients, they were used in small quantities as texture modifiers. They are now being used on a wider scale to replace fat. You can find such substitutes in cream dressings, candies, tinned meats, salad dressings, frozen desserts, spreads and dips, bakery and pastry products, prepared foods, etc.

There are many unanswered questions. If an individual decides to substitute half the fat he usually eats with some of these new fats, what will the cumulative effects be? Can these substitutes be eaten by every-body, or should they be reserved for certain groups of individuals? Substitutes such as Olestra are not digested. But what happens if minute amounts regularly pass through the digestive tract and into the bloodstream? Are there any risks of toxicity? Other substitutes are only partially digested; how will they affect the availability of fat-soluble vitamins A, D, E, and K, or the absorption of essential fatty acids, or certain medications?

We don't really know the long-term effects of a different intesti-nal flora on the synthesis of vitamin K, biotin, and other fatty acids. We do know, however, that these undigested substitutes can affect the flora and, can have a laxative effect or even cause an intestinal blockage. Can we connect the presence of these new fats to the intestinal problems some children are having? Should labels carry a warning or suggest a limited intake?

We would like to see these new fats help people reduce their fat intake and reach a healthful weight, but do we really know their long-term effect on total food intake? Do fat substitutes react the same way as sugar substitutes? In the United States, consumers are eating four times the amount of sugar substitutes they were taking in 1975, but they are also eating more sugar and still gaining weight. Will these fat substitutes be added to the actual fat intake instead of replacing them?

While they may think they are cutting down on fat and choles-terol, some people may actually be eating an overload of fat substitutes without knowing if there is any hope of a reduction in blood cholesterol.

> *The whole area of fat substitutes remains controversial, and we cannot recommend them as good fats.*

9

Doing It the Healthier Way

Follow the new golden rule and think *quality* when you choose fats at the grocery store, select items from a restaurant menu, and cook meals. Think *quantity* if you need to lose weight or have other health problems.

When you shop
Look for good fats such as:

- Extra-virgin olive oil or cold-pressed canola oil for your salad dressings and everyday cooking.
- Cold-pressed hazelnut oil to incorporate in salad dressings on party nights.
- Cold-pressed linseed oil for special uses.
- Almonds and walnuts for healthy snacks.
- Fish and seafood for good sources of omega-3 fatty acids.
- Tofu, soybeans, leafy green vegetables, and broccoli for extra omega-3s.
- Whole grains or whole-grain cereal products such as brown rice, whole-grain breads, and pasta to round up your supply of omega-6 fatty acids.

Ration your servings of meat, poultry, and cheese to limit the total amount of saturated fat.

Choose low-fat milk, low-fat fresh cheese (cottage, ricotta), and low-fat yogurt to get all the calcium and vitamins but little saturated fat.

Limit the bad fats and eliminate foods that contain hydrogenated and *trans*-fatty acids such as regular margarines, fried foods, chips, processed peanut butter, and crackers (see page 37 for more).

The following food lists show how easy it is to do it the healthier way. The first list (Table 16) is planned around *good* fats, the second (Table 17) is planned around *bad* fats. Making good choices does not only ensure quality but can provide an important reduction in quantity, 39 versus 133 grams of fat per day, a difference that can help you lose weight, if you wish to do so.

Table 16 Good choices		
FOOD GROUP		GRAMS OF FAT
CEREAL	1 homemade muffin	3.9 🍎
PRODUCTS	3 slices of whole-grain bread	1.5 🍎
	250 ml/1 cup brown rice	1.8 🍎
	1 bowl of bran cereal	1.4 🍎
VEGETABLES	1 baked potato	0.2 🍎
AND FRUITS	250 ml/1 cup broccoli or cauliflower	0.2 🍎
	1/4 avocado	7.5 🍎
	1 green salad, romaine lettuce	0.2 🍎
	1 glass of orange juice	0.2 🍎
	1 bowl of strawberries	0.3 🍎
MILK PRODUCTS	1 large glass of 1% milk	2.5 –
	1 bowl of 1.5% yogurt	2.0 –
	1 scoop of iced milk	3.0 –
MEATS AND	90 g/3 oz of grilled cod	4.5 🍎
SUBSTITUTES	250 ml/1 cup of cooked beans	1.3 🍎
FAT	10 ml/2 tsp of olive oil	9.0 🍎
DAILY TOTAL		39.5 grams

🍎   Food contains good fat
Ø   Food contains bad fat
Ø 🍎 Food contains both good and bad fat
–   Food contains neither good nor bad fat

Table 17 Poor choices		
FOOD GROUP		GRAMS OF FAT
GRAIN PRODUCTS	1 croissant	12.0 Ø
	8 whole-wheat crackers	6.2 Ø
	250 ml egg noodles	2.5 –
	4 cookies	6.8 Ø
VEGETABLES AND FRUITS	1 serving of french fries	10.0 Ø
	1 pastry filled with broccoli or cauliflower	17.0 Ø
	1 green salad, iceberg letuce	0.1 🍎
	1 glass of orange juice	0.2 🍎
	1 wedge of apple pie	13.1 Ø
MILK PRODUCTS	1 large glass of homo milk	8.6 –
	1 bowl of 3.25% yogurt	4.2 –
	1 scoop of ice cream	12.5 –
MEATS AND SUBSTITUTES	90 g breaded fish sticks	7.5 🍎 Ø
	250 ml meat sauce	10.2 –
FAT	15 ml margarine	11.0 Ø
	15 ml Italian salad dressing	10.3 🍎
DAILY TOTAL		132.2 grams

🍎   Food contains good fat
Ø   Food contains bad fat
Ø 🍎   Food contains both good and bad fat
–   Food contains neither good nor bad fat

In the kitchen
Cooking with good fats and decreasing the total quantity of all fats can help you become healthier without losing a gram of pleasure. One idea will give rise to another. You'll see!

For baked goods such as **cookies**, use nonfat or low-fat plain yogurt, canola oil, egg whites, cake flour, brown sugar, fruit purées, and more spices.

For **muffins**, use two egg whites for every whole egg; use canola oil instead of butter or margarine. Even if cold-pressed, canola oil will not reach high temperatures (not more than 87°C, or 190°F) in the oven.

Nothing comparable to frying temperatures.

For **pies**, eliminate one of the crusts in a double-crust pie, cut down on the butter, and switch to canola oil for the pastry. For one crust, combine 40 ml (3 tbsp) skim milk with 60 ml (4 tbsp) oil and blend with 265 ml (1 tbsp more than one cup) of whole-wheat pastry flour directly in the pie plate with fingertips or a fork. Or prepare a light quiche and forget the crust; it's the filling that has all the flavor!

For **cheesecake**, mix whole-grain cereal crumbs with hazelnut oil for the crust. For the filling, reduce the number of egg yolks and add extra egg whites; replace the regular cream cheese with a combination of low-fat cream cheese and low-fat yogurt, or use yogurt cheese.

Prepare **yogurt cheese** with low-fat plain yogurt. Line a colander with a double thickness of cheesecloth. Set over a large bowl. Spoon in yogurt, cover with plastic wrap, and refrigerate overnight. Transfer the cheese to a separate container. Discard the liquid. Yogurt cheese can be stored, covered, in the refrigerator for up to one week. Six cups of yogurt make about two cups of yogurt cheese.

For **phyllo pastry**, replace melted butter between layers with a mixture of egg whites and olive oil; lightly coat each sheet of phyllo.

On breakfast foods such as **toast**, forget the butter or the margarine and try applesauce, honey, a sliced banana, or special toppings such as fruit butters. To prepare, chop fresh, unpeeled apple or pear or dried fruit and slowly cook in apple juice, cider, water, or tea until very soft. Press the fruit through a sieve to remove the seeds and skins. Sweeten with honey or maple syrup. Add spices and return the purée to the stove; slowly simmer into a smooth, thick spread. Store in the refrigerator for as long as two weeks or in the freezer for up to six months.

If your cholesterol is too high but you can't live without fat on your toast, mix 125 ml (1/2 cup) of butter with 125 ml (1/2 cup) of cold-pressed canola or hazelnut oil; keep in the refrigerator and spread lightly on toast on Sundays!

Prepare **french toast** with egg whites, skim milk, and low-fat yogurt, and use a teaspoon of canola oil in a nonstick pan for every four slices.

Instead of frying **pancakes**, bake them. Use more egg whites than yolks, and use low-fat milk, whole-wheat flour, and vanilla. Bake at 425°F on a nonstick skillet for 15 to 20 minutes.

For **sandwiches**, use low-fat cheese or low-fat mayonnaise instead of butter or margarine. Try Dijon mustard on one side and plain yogurt or yogurt cheese on the other. This idea is especially interesting with chicken or turkey.

For a super sandwhich filled with *good* fat, mash a ripe avocado, sprinkle with a little lemon juice, and spread on whole-wheat pita bread or on a whole-grain bun instead of butter. Cover with slices of tomato and tuna.

For delicious **sauces**, thicken with garlic purée (garlic and chicken stock cooked together and blended until smooth), or mushroom purée instead of egg yolk, which is rich in saturated fat. Prolonged cooking can improve the taste.

To make a **white bechamel sauce**, use the *beurre manié* technique instead of preparing a roux with cooked fat. Mix together in a small bowl flour and olive or canola oil; incorporate this paste into the heated liquid and stir until thickened. To improve the flavor of the sauce, use part vegetable or chicken broth, part low-fat milk instead of milk alone.

To make **fry-a-like foods**, use bread crumbs mixed with finely chopped almonds or sesame seeds and fresh herbs; dip pieces of skin-free chicken breast or fresh fish in low-fat yogurt, then roll in breading. Bake on a lightly oiled cookie sheet or in a Pyrex dish at 200° to 225°C (400° to 450°F).

Oven-fry potatoes with unpeeled, scrubbed potatoes cut in pieces and lightly coated with a mixture of extra-virgin olive oil (30 ml, or 2 tbsp of oil, for 3 large potatoes), paprika, salt and pepper. Roast on a slightly oiled baking sheet, at 225°C (450°F) for 10 to 15 minutes, until brown.

For **salads**, sprinkle ripe tomato slices with balsamic vinegar; forget the oil-based dressing — the flavor of balsamic vinegar is absolutely exquisite! Sprinkle with chives if desired.

Prepare a **salad dressing** with half extra-virgin olive oil and half balsamic vinegar, a little Dijon mustard, and salt and pepper to taste; this recipe allows you reduce the usual proportion of oil and increase the flavor.

For **eggplant**, brush thin slices with a few drops of olive oil and a little crushed garlic; season and broil under the grill instead of cooking in a saucepan with loads of oil.

In restaurants

Whether you eat in a fast-food chain or an elegant five-star restaurant you can easily choose *good* fats and avoid excessive quantities.

To prove the point and help you do so, we have elaborated and evaluated eight daily menus corresponding to different lifestyles and budgets.

Four of these menus supply from 78 to 105 grams of fat per day; *bad* fats are frequent. The other four supply between 28 and 46 grams of fat, and *good* fats are well represented.

The secret does not lie in which restaurant you go to but in the foods you choose. And the pleasure of eating has no connection with the quantity of fat on the plate.

According to our new golden rule, foods that contain the monounsaturates, the alpha-linolenic, and omega-3 fatty acids are considered sources of *good* fats, while foods that contain hydrogenated fats or fried fats are considered sources of *bad* fats.

MENU 1
Eating in Fast-food Restaurants — Poor Choices

	Calories (cal)	Fat (g)	Rating
BREAKFAST			
Mcmuffin, sausages, and eggs	415	25	Ø
coffee with 10% cream (15 ml/1 tbsp)	19	2	–
LUNCH			
chicken nuggets	280	20	Ø
fries, small portion	240	12	Ø
diet cola	0	0	–
apple turnover	280	15	Ø
SUPPER			
pizza, medium (1 slice)	295	15	–
diet cola	0	0	–
SNACK			
vanilla ice-cream cone	140	4	–
TOTAL	1669	93	

Ø   source of bad fats
🍎   source of good fats
–   neither good nor bad fats

MENU 2
Eating in Fast-food Restaurants — Better Choices

	Calories (cal)	Fat (g)	Rating
BREAKFAST			
orange juice	80	0.2	🍎
cereal with nuts	100	1.3	🍎
2% milk (125 ml/1/2 cup)	64	2.5	–
whole-grain bread, toasted (2 slices)	132	1.2	🍎
butter (5 g/1 tsp)	36	4	–
coffee, black	0	0	–
LUNCH			
chili	220	7	🍎
small baked potato	135	0.2	🍎
garden salad	70	2	🍎
Italian salad dressing (15 ml/1 tbsp)	93	10.3	🍎
2% milk	110	4	–
cantaloup	20	0.2	🍎
SUPPER			
seafood pizza, medium (1 slice)	306	7	🍎
coffee with 2% milk	13	0.5	–
apple (whole)	81	0.5	🍎
SNACK			
frozen yogurt cone, medium size	126	1.1	–
TOTAL	1586	40.9	

Ø source of bad fats
🍎 source of good fats
– neither good nor bad fats

MENU 3
Eating at Home — Poor Choices

	Calories (cal)	Fat (g)	Rating
BREAKFAST			
Harvest Crunch cereal (100 ml/1/3 cup)	200	9	Ø
whole milk (125 ml/1/2 cup)	80	4	–
coffee with cream	18	2	–
LUNCH			
spaghetti with lean meat sauce	173	3	–
refined pasta, cooked (250 ml/1 cup)	164	1	–
salad (lettuce, spinach, tomatoes, cucumbers)	36	0.2	🍎
mayonnaise	86	10	–
commercial muffin	225	11	Ø
SUPPER			
trout (100 g/3 oz) fried in	216	13	🍎
margarine (10 ml/2 tsp)	67	9	Ø
baked potato	110	0.2	🍎
sour cream (30 ml/2 tbsp)	47	4	–
green beans (125 ml/1/2 cup)	23	0.2	🍎
with margarine (5 ml/1 tsp)	36	4	Ø
SNACK			
Quaker Dipps granola bar (melted chocolate and peanut butter)	175	10	Ø
TOTAL	1616	82.6	

Ø   source of bad fats
🍎   source of good fats
–   neither good nor bad fats

MENU 4
Eating at Home — Better Choices

	Calories (cal)	Fat (g)	Rating
BREAKFAST			
half grapefruit	37	0.1	🍎
homemade müesli cereal	217	6	🍎
(225 ml/3/4 cup) (oats, lemon, milk, maple syrup, almonds, apples)			
1% yogurt (60 ml/4 tbsp), added to cereal	35	1	–
milk partially skimmed (250 ml/1 cup)	110	3	–
coffee with cream	18	2	–
LUNCH			
spaghetti and tomato sauce with tofu	170	9	🍎
whole-wheat pasta, cooked (250 ml/1 cup)	160	1	🍎
salad (lettuce, spinach, tomatoes, cucumbers)	36	0.2	🍎
extra-virgin olive oil (5 ml/1 tsp)	40	5	🍎
balsamic vinegar (5 ml/1 tsp)	1	0	–
seven grain bread (1 slice)	80	1	🍎
fruit salad (250 ml/1 cup)	121	0.1	🍎
SUPPER			
trout (100 g/3 oz), braised	216	13	🍎
baked potato (1 small)	110	0.2	🍎
yogurt (30 ml/2 tbsp)	18	0.3	
steamed broccoli (250 ml/1 cup) with lemon	47	0.3	🍎
homemade muffin	136	4	🍎
SNACK			
kefir or natural 1% yogurt (125 ml/1/2 cup)	80	2	–
fresh strawberries, sliced (125 m/1/2 cup)	24	0.3	🍎
TOTAL	1638	46.3	

Ø   source of bad fats
🍎   source of good fats
–   neither good nor bad fats

MENU 5
Eating at Home and at a Restaurant — Poor Choices

	Calories (cal)	Fat (g)	Rating
BREAKFAST (at home)			
bacon slices (2)	72	7	–
fried eggs in margarine	115	10	Ø
whole-wheat bread	8	1	●
margarine (5 ml/1 tsp)	36	4	Ø
LUNCH (at a restaurant)			
chicken salad with cheese & Caesar dressing	550	40	–
fries	290	15	Ø
diet cola	0	0	–
SUPPER (at home)			
frozen dinner: cannelloni with cheese	260	12	–
10% yogurt (125 ml/1/2 cup)	284	13	–
SNACK			
cookie (1)	49	2	Ø
TOTAL	1616	103	

Ø source of bad fats
● source of good fats
– neither good nor bad fats

MENU 6
Eating at Home and at a Restaurant — Better Choices

	Calories (cal)	Fat (g)	Rating
BREAKFAST (at home)			
apple juice (125 ml/1/2 cup)	62	0.1	🍎
boiled egg	79	6	–
7-grain bread	80	1	🍎
butter (5 ml/1 tsp)	36	4	–
1% milk (250 ml/1 cup)	110	3	–
LUNCH (at a restaurant)			
chicken breast in salad	222	2	–
herb salad dressing (15 ml/1 tbsp)	71	7.9	🍎
whole-wheat bread (1 slice)	80	1	🍎
fresh fruit cocktail	95	0.1	🍎
SUPPER (at home)			
frozen dinner: lasagne with zucchini	260	7	–
7-grain bread	80	1	🍎
1% yogurt	110	1.6	–
SNACK			
nuts and dried fruit (30 ml/2 tbsp)	95	2	🍎
1% milk (250 ml/1 cup)	110	3	–
TOTAL	1490	39.7	

Ø   source of bad fats
🍎 source of good fats
–   neither good nor bad fats

MENU 7
Fine Dining — Poor Choices

	Calories (cal)	Fat (g)	Rating
BREAKFAST			
grapefruit juice (125 ml/1/2 cup)	51	0.1	🍎
warm croissant	235	12	Ø
butter (5 ml/1 tsp)	35	4	–
coffee with cream (30 ml/2 tbsp)	56	6	–
LUNCH			
Dubarry soup (200 ml/3/4 cup) (*cream of cauliflower*)	177	15	–
crusty bun	156	1.6	–
cheese platter (60 g)	211	18.5	–
SUPPER			
roast loin of veal (60 g/2 oz), (*veal, butter, white wine*)	362	20	–
mushroom sauce (50 ml/1/4 cup) (*butter, flour, mushrooms, egg yolks, cream, stock, nutmeg*)	73	2	–
potatoes à la Dauphinoise (85 ml/1/3 c) (*potatoes, onion, gruyère cheese, cream*)	90	7	–
Vichy carrots (125 ml/1/2 cup) (*carrots, butter, parsley*)	86	6	–
fresh strawberries (125 ml/1/2 cup)	24	0.3	🍎
custard (65 ml/1/4 cup) (*icing sugar, egg yolks, milk, vanilla*)	98	4	–
TOTAL	1624	102.5	

Ø   source of bad fats
🍎   source of good fats
–   neither good nor bad fats

MENU 8
Fine Dining — Better Choices

	Calories (cal)	Fat (g)	Rating
BREAKFAST			
half grapefruit	37	0.1	🍎
bran muffin	136	4	🍎
cottage cheese (125 ml/1/2 cup)	89	1	–
coffee with 2% milk	16	0.6	–
LUNCH			
tomato and basil soup (*tomatoes, onion, celery, olive oil, basil, garlic, bouquet garni, salt, pepper*)	73	3	🍎
vegetable bundles and filet of sole Regence (*filets of sole, shrimp, carrots, celery root, zucchini, spinach, green beans, shallots, mushrooms, white wine, mussels, spices*)	233	2	🍎
whole-grain bread (1 slice)	80	1	🍎
butter (5 ml/1 tsp)	36	4	–
light strawberry mille-feuille (*yogurt, flour, oil, milk, sugar, strawberries, lemon mint, corn starch, salt*)	164	2	–
tea	0	0	–
SUPPER			
garden tofu lasagne (*tofu, carrots, turnip, celeriac, potatoes, zucchini, spinach, corn starch, skim milk, chicken stock, egg white, spices*)	293	6	🍎
whole-grain bread (1 slice)	80	1	🍎
kiwi sherbet (*kiwis, strawberries, orange, lemon, sugar*)	200	1	🍎
SNACK			
1% milk (250 ml/1 cup)	105	3	–
TOTAL	1542	28.7	

Ø   source of bad fats
🍎   source of good fats
–   neither good nor bad fats

APPENDIX

Fat Content of Some Foods

FAT CONTENT OF SOME FOODS				
	PORTION		FAT	RATING
MEATS	Imperial	metric	(g)	
Beef, cooked without fat				
stew, lean	3 oz	90 g	9	–
steak, regular	3 oz	90 g	9	–
steak, lean	3 oz	90 g	6	–
ground beef, regular	3 oz	90 g	17	–
ground beef, lean	3 oz	90 g	13	–
rib roast, regular	3 oz	90 g	18	–
rib roast, lean	3 oz	90 g	10	–
rump roast, regular	3 oz	90 g	10	–
rump roast, lean	3 oz	90 g	7	–
Lamb, cooked without fat				
leg, regular	3 oz	90 g	16	–
leg, lean	3 oz	90 g	6	–
chop, regular	3 oz	90 g	35	–
chop, lean	3 oz	90 g	7	–
Pork, cooked without fat				
tenderloin, lean	3 oz	90 g	4	–
loin, regular	3 oz	90 g	19	–
loin, lean	3 oz	90 g	9	–
rump (leg), regular	3 oz	90 g	14	–
rump (leg), lean	3 oz	90 g	7	–
Veal, cooked without fat				
chop or sirloin steak	3 oz	90 g	12	–
Liver, cooked without fat				
veal	3 oz	90 g	4	–
chicken	3 oz	90 g	4	–
pork	3 oz	90 g	4	–
beef	3 oz	90 g	4	–

Ø   source of bad fats
🍎   source of good fats
–   neither good nor bad fats

FAT CONTENT OF SOME FOODS				
	PORTION		FAT	RATING
MEATS	Imperial	metric	(g)	
Delicatessen				
2 frankfurters	1 oz	30 g	10	–
1 smoked sausage (beef/pork)	1.3 oz	37 g	11	–
1 smoked sausage (turkey)	1.3 oz	37 g	7	–
1 slice of cooked ham	1 oz	30 g	3	–
1 slice of salami	3/4 oz	22 g	4	–
1 slice of bologna	3/4 oz	23 g	6	–
3 slices of blood sausage	3 oz	90 g	30	–
liver pâté	3 tbsp	45 ml	12	–
bacon, back	2 slices	50 g	4	–
bacon, strips	3 slices	20 g	9	–
Chicken and turkey				
chicken, white meat, without skin	3 oz	90 g	4	–
chicken, brown meat, without skin	3 oz	90 g	9	–
chicken, white meat with skin	3 oz	90 g	7	–
turkey, white meat, without skin	3 oz	90 g	3	–
turkey, brown meat, without skin	3 oz	90 g	6	–

Ø   source of bad fats
🍎 source of good fats
–   neither good nor bad fats

FAT CONTENT OF SOME FOODS				
	PORTION		FAT	RATING
FISH AND SEAFOOD	Imperial	metric	(g)	
Fish				
salmon, trout, mackerel	3 oz	90 g	12	🍎
sardines, white fish	3 oz	90 g	12	🍎
herring	3 oz	90 g	12	🍎
flounder	3 oz	90 g	8	🍎
halibut, pollock	3 oz	90 g	5	🍎
pickerel, yellow perch, smelt	3 oz	90 g	2	🍎
cod, sole, skate	3 oz	90 g	1	🍎
tuna, canned in water	3 oz	90 g	1	🍎
tuna, canned in oil, strained	3 oz	90 g	7	🍎
anchovy	1 oz	26 g	2	🍎
Shellfish and seafood				
squid	3 oz	90 g	2	🍎
caviar	1 tbsp	15 ml	2	🍎
crab	3 oz	90 g	2	🍎
shrimps	3 oz	90 g	1	🍎
frog legs	3 oz	90 g	2	🍎
snails	3 oz	90 g	1	🍎
lobster	3 oz	90 g	1	🍎
oysters	3 oz	90 g	2	🍎
mussels, clams	3 oz	90 g	2	🍎
scallops	3 oz	90 g	1	🍎

Ø　source of bad fats
🍎　source of good fats
−　neither good nor bad fats

FAT CONTENT OF SOME FOODS				
	PORTION		FAT	RATING
EGGS, LEGUMES, SEEDS NUTS, AND ALTERNATIVES	Imperial	metric	(g)	
1 large egg		50 g	6	–
1 egg yolk		17 g	6	–
1 egg white		33 g	traces	–
lentils, split peas, cooked	1 cup	250 ml	1	🍎
white or red beans, cooked	1 cup	250 ml	1	🍎
chick peas, cooked	1 cup	250 ml	4	🍎
soybeans, cooked	1 cup	250 ml	11	🍎
soya milk	1 cup	250 ml	5	🍎
tempeh (soybeans, fermented)	1 cup	250 ml	13	🍎
tofu silken	1/2 cup	125 ml	6	🍎
tofu firm	1/2 cup	125 ml	11	🍎
almonds and walnuts	1/4 cup	60 ml	20	🍎
peanuts and hazelnuts	1/4 cup	60 ml	19	🍎
pecan and pistachio	1/4 cup	60 ml	19	🍎
pine nuts	1/4 cup	60 ml	22	–
cashews	1/4 cup	60 ml	17	🍎
brazil nuts	1/4 cup	60 ml	25	🍎
coconut	1/4 cup	60 ml	7	–
peanut butter, regular	1 tbsp	15 ml	8	Ø
peanut butter, natural	1 tbsp	15 ml	8	🍎
almond butter, natural	1 tbsp	15 ml	10	🍎
sesame seed butter (tahini)	1 tbsp	15 ml	8	–
pumpkin seeds	1/4 cup	60 ml	14	–
sesame seeds	1/4 cup	60 ml	22	–
sunflower seeds	1/4 cup	60 ml	19	–

Ø   source of bad fats
🍎   source of good fats
–   neither good nor bad fats

FAT CONTENT OF SOME FOODS				
	PORTION		FAT	RATING
DAIRY PRODUCTS	Imperial	metric	(g)	
Milk				
whole milk (3.25%)	1 cup	250 ml	9	–
2% milk	1 cup	250 ml	5	–
1% milk	1 cup	250 ml	3	–
skim milk	1 cup	250 ml	traces	–
powder skim milk	1 tbsp	15 ml	traces	–
soya milk	1 cup	250 ml	5	🍎
Cheese, firm,				
semi-firm or melted				
with 35% b.f.	1.5 oz	45 g	16	–
gruyère	1.5 oz	45 g	16	–
blue	1.5 oz	45 g	16	–
havarti	1.5 oz	45 g	16	–
with 30% b.f.				
cheddar	1.5 oz	45 g	14	–
colby	1.5 oz	45 g	14	–
monterey	1.5 oz	45 g	14	–
münster	1.5 oz	45 g	14	–
parmesan	1.5 oz	45 g	14	–
roquefort	1.5 oz	45 g	14	–
with 28% b.f.				
brie	1.5 oz	45 g	13	–
edam	1.5 oz	45 g	13	–
emmental	1.5 oz	45 g	13	–
gouda	1.5 oz	45 g	13	–
limburger	1.5 oz	45 g	13	–
provolone	1.5 oz	45 g	13	–
romano	1.5 oz	45 g	13	–

Ø source of bad fats
🍎 source of good fats
– neither good nor bad fats

FAT CONTENT OF SOME FOODS				
	PORTION		FAT	RATING
DAIRY PRODUCTS	Imperial	metric	(g)	
with 25% b.f.				
camembert	1.5 oz	45 g	12	–
feta	1.5 oz	45 g	12	–
mozzarella	1.5 oz	45 g	12	–
neufchatel	1.5 oz	45 g	12	–
swiss	1.5 oz	45 g	12	–
tilsit	1.5 oz	45 g	12	–
with 20% b.f.				
Cracker Barrel	1.5 oz	45 g	7	–
baron	1.5 oz	45 g	7	–
goat cheese	1.5 oz	45 g	7	–
with 15% b.f.				
brick skim	1.5 oz	45 g	9	–
emmental type	1.5 oz	45 g	9	–
goat cheese	1.5 oz	45 g	9	–
havarti, part skim	1.5 oz	45 g	9	–
brie	1.5 oz	45 g	9	–
jarlsberg	1.5 oz	45 g	9	–
mozzarella, part skim	1.5 oz	45 g	9	–
with 7% or 8% b.f.				
allegro	1.5 oz	45 g	3	–
danbo	1.5 oz	45 g	3	–
la vache qui rit	1.5 oz	45 g	3	–
Cottage cheese				
creamed (4% b.f.)	1/2 cup	125 ml	4	–
2% b.f.	1/2 cup	125 ml	2	–
1% b.f.	1/2 cup	125 ml	1	–
0.4% b.f.	1/2 cup	125 ml	traces	–
Fromagisoy				
(melted tofu cheese type)				
light (reduced in fat)	1.5 oz	45 g	traces	🍎
regular	1.5 oz	45 g	7	🍎

Ø source of bad fats
🍎 source of good fats — neither good nor bad fats

FAT CONTENT OF SOME FOODS				
	PORTION		FAT	RATING
DAIRY PRODUCTS	Imperial	metric	(g)	
Yogurt				
fruit, 4.5% b.f.	3/4 cup	175 ml	8	–
plain, 3.9% b.f.	3/4 cup	175 ml	7	–
plain, 3.2% b.f.	3/4 cup	175 ml	6	–
plain, 3.1% b.f.	3/4 cup	175 ml	6	–
plain, 2% b.f.	3/4 cup	175 ml	4	–
fruit or plain, 1% b.f.	3/4 cup	175 ml	2	–
fruit or plain, 0.1% b.f.	3/4 cup	175 ml	traces	–
Other milk fermented products				
Astro yogurt and granola, 1.3% b.f.	1/2 cup	125 mL	2	–
Biobest Plus, 1.2% b.f.	3/4 cup	175 ml	2	–
Yop, 1.7% b.f.	3/4 cup	175 ml	3	–
Yop, 1.0% b.f.	3/4 cup	175 ml	2	–
Ice cream and frozen deserts				
ice cream, regular, 10% b.f.	1 cup	250 ml	15	–
ice milk, 4% b.f.	1 cup	250 ml	6	–
frozen yogurt, 2.7% b.f.	1 cup	250 ml	5	–
sherbet, 2% b.f.	1 cup	250 ml	4	–
sherbet, nonfat, 0.1% b.f.	1 cup	250 ml	traces	–
Cream				
cream, 35% B.F.	1 tbsp	15 ml	5	–
cream, 15% B.F.	1 tbsp	15 ml	2	–
cream, 10% B.F.	1 tbsp	15 ml	1.5	–
sour cream, 14% B.F.	1 tbsp	15 ml	3	–
light sour cream, 5% B.F.	1 tbsp	15 mL	1	–
FRUITS AND VEGETABLES				
all fruits but avocado	–	traces		&#x1F34E;
avocado from California	1/2	88 g	15	&#x1F34E;
from Florida	1/2	150 g	14	&#x1F34E;
vegetables	–	–	traces	&#x1F34E;

Ø   source of bad fats

🍎   source of good fats

–   neither good nor bad fats

FAT CONTENT OF SOME FOODS				
	PORTION		FAT	RATING
OILS AND FATS	Imperial	metric	(g)	
oil: olive, canola, hazelnut	1 tbsp	15 ml	14	🍎
butter, regular	1 tbsp	15 ml	11	−
butter, calorie reduced, 50% less fat	1 tbsp	15 mL	6	−
margarine	1 tbsp	15 ml	11	Ø
mayonnaise, regular	1 tbsp	15 ml	11	Ø
salad dressing, light	1 tbsp	15 ml	5	−
salad dressing, with *good* fat	1 tbsp	15 ml	6	🍎
GRAIN, BREAD AND PASTA				
white or whole-wheat bread	1 slice		1	🍎 Ø
some whole-grain breads	1 slice		1	🍎 Ø
some whole-wheat breads	1 slice		3	🍎 Ø
tortilla	1		1	🍎 Ø
pita bread	1		1	🍎 Ø
bagel	1		2	🍎 Ø
Danish	1		2	Ø
hot-dog bun	1		2	Ø
hamburger bun	1		2	Ø
oatmeal, cooked	1 cup	250 ml	3	🍎
rice or barley, cooked	1 cup	250 ml	1	🍎
pasta, cooked	1 cup	250 ml	1	🍎
pancakes, 1 medium			2	−
doughnut, 1			8	Ø
croissant, 1			12	Ø
muffin made with *good* fat, 1 small			4	🍎
muffin commercial, 1 large			9	Ø
English muffin , 1			1	−
dry cereals	1 oz	30 g	1	🍎 Ø
granola type cereal	1 oz	30 g	6	🍎 Ø

Ø   source of bad fats   🍎 Ø   both good and bad fats
🍎   source of good fats   −   neither good nor bad fats

FAT CONTENT OF SOME FOODS				
	PORTION		FAT	RATING
PASTRY AND COOKIES	Imperial	metric	(g)	
cake with icing	2 oz	60 g	12	Ø
cheesecake	3 oz	90 g	18	Ø
fruit pie	5 oz	150 g	18	Ø
chocolate-chip cookie, 1			4	Ø
peanut-butter cookie, 1			4	Ø
arrowroot cookie, 1			1	Ø
melba toast, saltine, 1			traces	Ø
rice cake, 1			traces	
FAST FOOD				
chips, 30			21	Ø
pretzels	1 oz	30 g	1	Ø
popcorn without butter	1 cup	250 ml	traces	–
popcorn with butter	1 cup	250 ml	4	–
chocolate bar	1.65 oz	54 g	15	Ø
fried chicken	3 oz	90 g	15	Ø
fish sticks	3 oz	90 g	14	Ø
pizza with cheese, 1 slice			7	–
pizza with pepperoni, 1 slice			9	–
hot dog (bun and frankfurter)		90 g	14	Ø
hamburger (bun and meat)		90 g	11	Ø
french fries	3 oz	85 g	14	Ø
milkshake	1 cup	250 ml	6	–

Ø   source of bad fats
🍎   source of good fats
–   neither good nor bad fats

For more information:

• *Health and Welfare Canada.*
  Nutritive Value of Some Common Foods.
  Ottawa: Government of Canada, 1988.

• *Pennington, J. A. T.*
  Food Values of Portions Commonly
  Used. *Bowes and Church's, 1989.*

BIBLIOGRAPHY

CHAPTER 1

On Actual and Potential Essential Fatty Acid Deficiency

Cunnane, S. C., et al. "Essential fatty acid and lipid profiles in plasma and erythrocytes in patients with multiple sclerosis," in *American Journal of Clinical Nutrition*, 50 (1989): 801–6.

Hennig, B., and B. A. Walkins. "Linoleic acid and linolenic acid: effect on permeability properties of culture endothelial cells monolayers," in *American Journal of Clinical Nutrition*, 49 (1989): 301–15.

Holman, R. T., et al. "Deficiency of essential fatty acids and membrane fluidity during pregnancy and lactation," in *Proceedings of the National Academy of Sciences*, 88 (1991): 4835–39.

Holman, R. T., and S. B. Johnson. "Essential fatty acid deficiencies in man," in *Dietary Fats and Health*, Ed. by E. G. Perkins, and W. J. Visek. Champaign, Ill: American Oil Chemists' Society, 1983: 247–66.

Swank, R. H., and A. Grimsgaard. "Multiple sclerosis: the lipid relationship," in *American Journal of Clinical Nutrition*, 48 (1988): 1387–93.

Ziboh, V. A. "Implications of dietary oils and polyunsaturated fatty acids in the management of cutaneous disorders," in *Archives of Dermatology*, 125 (1989): 241–45.

On the Needs of the Fetus for Essential Fatty Acids

Crawford, M. A. "The role of essential fatty acids in neural development: implications for perinatal nutrition," in *American Journal of Clinical Nutrition*, 57 (suppl.) (1993): 703S–10S.

Nettleton, J. A. "Are n-3 fatty acids essential nutrients for fetal and infant development?" in *Journal of the American Dietetic Association,* 93 (1993): 58–64.

Ricardo, D., et al. "Effect of dietary omega-3 fatty acids on retinal function of very-low-birth-weight neonates," in *Pediatric Research,* 28 (1990): 485–92.

On Essential Fatty Acids and Adequate Transport of Cholesterol and Other Fats

Levy, E., et al. "Lipoprotein abnormalities associated with cholesteryl ester transfer activity in cystic fibrosis patients: the role of essential fatty acid deficiency," in *American Journal of Clinical Nutrition,* 57 (1993): 573–9.

On Fat Content of Breast Milk

Makrides M., et al. "Fatty acid composition of brain, retina, and erythrocytes in breast- and formula-fed infants," in *American Journal of Clinical Nutrition,* 60 (1994): 189–94.

Innis, S. M. "Human milk and formula fatty acids," in *The Journal of Pediatrics,* 120 (1992): S56–61.

On Essential Fatty Acids; Their Derivatives and Health Implications

Batres-Cerezo, R., et al. "Studies of women eating diets with different fatty acids composition. III. Fatty acids and prostaglandins synthesis by platelets and cultured human endothelial cells," in *Journal of the American College of Nutrition,* 10 (1991): 327–39.

Crawford, M. A., et al. "Essential fatty acids and the vulnerability of the artery during growth," in *Postgraduate Medical Journal,* 54 (1978): 149–53.

Sinclair A., and R. Gibson. *Essential Fatty Acids and Eicosanoids.* Champaign, Ill: American Oil Chemist's Society, 1992.

On Optimal Health Depends on Optimal Ratio of the Two Essential Fatty Acids

Siguel, E., and R. H. Lerman. "Altered fatty acid metabolism in patients with angiographically documented coronary artery disease," in *Metabolism,* 43 (8) (1994): 982–93.

On Linoleic Acid and Ulcers

Grant, H. W. "Duodenal ulcer is associated with low dietary linoleic acid intake," in *Gut*, 31 (1990): 997–8.

Hollander, D., and A. Tarnawski. "Dietary essential fatty acids and the decline in peptic ulcer disease — a hypothesis," in *Gut*, 27 (1986): 239–42.

Kearney, J., et al. "Dietary intakes and adipose tissue levels of linoleic acid in peptic ulcer disease," in *British Journal of Nutrition*, 62 (1989): 699–706.

On Coronary Heart Disease and a New Form of Essential Fatty Acid Deficiency

Roberts, T. L., et al. "Linoleic acid and risk of sudden cardiac death," in *British Heart Journal*, 70 (6) (1993): 524–29.

Siguel, E. N., and R. H. Lerman. "Altered fatty acid metabolism in patient with angiographically documented coronary artery disease," in *Metabolism*, 43 (8) (1994): 982–93.

Emken, E. A. "Nutrition and biochemistry of trans and positional fatty acid isomers in hydrogenated oils," in *Annual Review of Nutrition*, 4 (1984): 339–76.

On the Elderly and a Deficiency in Essential Fatty Acids

Asciutti-Moura, L. S., et al. "Fatty acid composition of serum lipids and its relation to diet in an elderly institutionalized population," in *American Journal of Clinical Nutrition*, 48 (1988): 980–87.

Dillon, J. C. "Essential fatty acid in metabolism in the elderly: effects of dietary manipulation," in *Lipids in Modern Nutrition*. New York: Vevey/Raven Press, 1987.

On Modern Diseases and Deficiency in Essential Fatty Acids

Sinclair, H. M. "Deficiency of essential fatty acids and atherosclerosis, etcetera," in *Lancet*, 1956: 381–83.

On the Omega-3 Fatty Acids and the Treatment of Certain Illnesses

Benquet, C. Lecture given at the annual congress of ACFAS, *La Presse*, May 14, 1992.

Burr, M. L., et al. "Effects of changes in fat, fish, and fibre intakes on death and myocardial reinfarction: diet and reinfarction trial (DART)," in *Lancet*, (1989): 757–61.

de Lorgeril, M., et al. "Mediterranean alpha-linolenic acid rich diet in secondary prevention of coronary heart disease," in *Lancet*, 343 (1994): 1454–59.

Haglund, O. *Effects of fish oil on risk factors for cardiovascular disease*. Acta Universitatis Uppsaliensis, Comprehensive Summaries of Uppsala Dissertations from the Faculty of Medecine, 428 (1993).

Kelley, D. S., et al. "Dietary alpha-linolenic acid and immunocompetence in humans," in *American Journal of Clinical Nutrition*, 53 (1991): 40–46.

Lévy, E., et al. "Beneficial effects of fish-oil supplements on lipids, lipoproteins, and lipoprotein lipase in patients with glycogen storage disease, type-1," in *American Journal of Clinical Nutrition*, 57 (1993): 922–29.

Mantzioris E., et al. "Dietary substitution with an alpha-linolenic acid-rich vegetable oil increases eicosapentaenoic acids concentrations in tissues," in *American Journal of Clinical Nutrition*, 59 (1994): 1304–9.

Neilsen, G. L., et al. "The effects of dietary supplementation with rheumatoid arthritis: a randomized, double-blind trial," in *European Journal of Clinical Investigation*, 22 (1992): 687–91.

Rose, D. P., and J. M. Connolly. "Effects of dietary omega-3 fatty acids on human breast cancer growth and metastases in nude mice," in *Journal of the National Cancer Institute*, 85 (21) (1993): 1743–47.

Salomon, P., et al. "Treatment of ulcerative colitis with fish oil n-3-fatty acid: An open trial," in *Journal of Clinical Gastroenterology*, 12 (1990): 157–61.

Shahar E., et al. "Dietary n-3 polyunsaturated fatty acids and smoking–related chronic obstructive pulmonary disease," in *The New England Journal of Medecine*, 331 (4) (1994): 228–33.

On the Nutritional Value of Some Foods

Human Nutrition Information Service. *Composition of Foods. Handbook No. 8.* Washington: United States Department of Agriculture, 1976–86.

CHAPTER 2

On Canadian Statistics for Cardiovascular Disease

Heart and Stroke Foundation of Ontario. "Canadian statistics," *Statistics Canada*, 1993.

On Diet, Blood Cholesterol Level, and the Risk of Developing Cardiovascular Disease

Bang, H. O., et al. "Plasma lipid and lipoprotein pattern in Greenlandic west-coast Eskimos," in *Lancet*, 1 (1971): 1143–46.

Blankenhorn, D. H., et al. "The influence of diet on the appearance of new lesions in human coronary arteries," in *Journal of the American Medical Association*, 263 (1990): 1646–52.

———— "Dietary fat influences human coronary lesion formation," in *Circulation*, 76 (suppl. II) (1988): 11.

Grundy, S. M., and G. V. Vega. "Plasma cholesterol responsiveness to saturated fatty acids," in *American Journal of Clinical Nutrition*, 47 (1988): 822–24.

Kestin, M., I. L. Rouse, R. A. Correll, and P. Nestel. "Cardiovascular disease risk factors in free-living men: Comparison of two prudent diets, one based on lacto-ovo-vegetarianism and the other allowing lean meat," in *American Journal of Clinical Nutrition*, 50 (1989): 280–87.

Kinsella, J., et al. "Dietary n-3 polyunsaturated fatty acids and amelioration of cardiovascular disease: possible mechanisms," in *American Journal of Clinical Nutrition*, 52 (1990): 1–28.

Nordöy, A., et al. "Individual effects of dietary saturated fatty acids and fish oil on plasma lipids and lipoproteins in normal man," in *American Journal of Clinical Nutrition*, 57 (1993): 634–39.

Ramsay, L. E., et al. "Dietary reduction of serum cholesterol concentration: Time to think again," in *British Medical Journal*, 303 (1991): 953–7.

Health and Welfare Canada. *Promoting Heart Health in Canada: A Focus on Cholesterol*. Ottawa: Health and Welfare Canada, 1991.

Wenxun, F., et al. "Erythrocyte fatty acids, plasma lipids, and cardiovascular disease in rural China," in *American Journal of Clinical Nutrition*, 52 (1990): 1027–36.

Zsigmond, E., et al. "Changes in dietary lipid saturation modify fatty acid composition and high-density-lipoprotein binding of adipocyte plasma membrane," in *American Journal of Clinical Nutrition*, 52 (1990): 110–19.

On Highly Processed Fats and *Trans*-fatty Acids

Ascherio, A. L., et al. "*Trans*-fatty acids intake and risk of myocardial infarction," in *Circulation*, 89 (1) (1994): 94–101.

Hasegawa, K., et al. "Nutritional assessment trial (fatty acids in particular) in community health and nutrition in Japan," in *The Third International Congress on Essential Fatty Acids and Eicosanoids*. Champaign, Ill: American Oil Chemists' Society, 1992: 81–83

Hudgins, L. C., et al. "Correlation of isomeric fatty acids in human adipose tissue with clinical risk factors for cardiovascular disease," in *American Journal of Clinical Nutrition*, 53 (1991): 474–82.

Siguel E. N., et al. "*Trans*-fatty acids patterns in patients with angiographically documented coronary heart disease," in *American Journal of Cardiology*, 71 (1993): 916–20.

Troisi, R., et al. "*Trans*-fatty acid intake in relation to serum lipid concentrations in adult men," in *American Journal of Clinical Nutrition*, 56 (1992): 1019–24.

Willet, W. C., and A. Ascherio. "*Trans*-fatty acids: Are the effects only marginal?" in *American Journal of Public Health*, 84(5) (1994): 1–3.

Willett, W. C., et al. "Intake of *trans*-fatty acids and risk of coronary heart disease among women," in *Lancet*, 241 (1993): 581–85.

On Healthier Lifestyle Can Help a Majority of Patients with Blocked Arteries

Ornish, D., et al. "Adherence to lifestyle changes and reversal of coronary atherosclerosis," in *Circulation*, 80(4) (1989): 11–57.

────── "Can lifestyle changes reverse coronary heart disease?" in *Lancet*, 336 (1990): 129–33.

────── *Dr. Dean Ornish's Program for Reversing Heart Disease*, New York: Random House, 1990.

On Cancer Statistics

National Cancer Institute of Canada, "Canadian Cancer Statistics," *Statistics Canada, Provincial Cancer Registries, Health Canada*, 1994.

On Diet, Fat, and Cancer

Bravo, M. G., et al. "Effects of an eicosapentaenoic and docosahexaenoic acid concentrate on a human lung carcinoma grown in nude mice," in *Lipids*, 26 (1991): 866–870.

Burkitt, D. "An approach to the reduction of most western cancers: The failure of therapy to reduce disease," in *Archives in Surgery*, 126 (1991): 345–47.

Carroll, K. K. "Dietary fats and cancer," in *American Journal of Clinical Nutrition*, 53 (1991): 1064S–7S.

────── "Lipids and carcinogenesis," in *Journal of Environmental Pathology and Toxicology*, 3 (1980): 253–71.

Carroll, K. K., and M. B. Davidson. "The role of lipids in tumorigenesis," in *Molecular Interrelations of Nutrition and Cancer*, (1982): 231–244.

On Breast Cancer

Bennett, B. C., and D. Ingram. "Diet and female sex hormone concentrations: an intervention study for the type of fat consumed," in *American Journal of Clinical Nutrition*, 52 (1990): 808–12.

Boyar, A. P., et al. "Recommendations for the prevention of chronic disease: the application for breast disease," in *American Journal of Clinical Nutrition*, 48 (1988): 896–900.

Carroll, K. K., and G. J. Hopkins. "Dietary polyunsaturated fat versus saturated fat in relation to mammary carcinogenesis," in *Lipids*, 14(2) (1978): 155–58.

Davidson, M. B., and K. K. Carroll. "Inhibitory effect of a fat free diet of mammary carcinogenesis in rats," abstract, 1981.

Ewertz, M., and C. Gill. "Dietary factors and breast-cancer risk in Denmark," in *International Journal of Cancer*, 46 (1990): 779–84.

Hopkins, J. G., and K. K. Carroll. "Relations between amount and type of dietary fat in promotion of mammary carcinogenesis induced by 7,12 dimethylbenz(a)anthracene," in *Journal of the National Cancer Institute*, 62(4) (1979): 1009–12.

Howe, G. R., et al. "A cohort study of fat intake and risk of breast cancer," in *Journal of the National Cancer Institute*, 83 (1991): 336–40.

Knekt, P., et al. "Dietary fat and risk of breast cancer," in *American Journal of Clinical Nutrition*, 52 (1990): 903–8.

Ingram, D. M., et al. "Prolactin and breast cancer risk," in *Medical Journal of Australia*, 153 (1990): 469–73.

———— "The role of diet in the development of breast cancer, benign hyperplasia and fibrocystic disease of the breast," in *British Journal of Cancer*, 64 (1991): 187–91.

Riboli, E., et al. "Diet and bladder cancer in Spain: A multi-centre case-control study," in *International Journal of Cancer*, 49 (1991): 214–19.

Shun-Zang, Y., et al. "A Case-control study of dietary and nondietary risk factors for breast cancer in Shanghai," in *Cancer Research*, 50 (1990): 5017–21.

Visek, W. J. "Dietary fat and cancer." Paper presented at the XXIII International Congress of the Dairy Industry, Montreal, 1990.

Woods, M. N., et al. "Low-fat, high fiber and serum estrone sulfate in premenopausal women," in *American Journal of Clinical Nutrition*, 49 (1989): 1179–83.

On Colon Cancer

Allinger, U. G., et al. "Shift from a mixed to a lactovegetarian diet: influence on acidic lipids in fecal water. A potential risk factor for colon cancer," in *American Journal of Clinical Nutrition*, 50 (1989): 992–96.

Benito, E. O., et al. "A population-based case-control study of colorectal cancer in Majorca. 1. Dietary factors," in *International Journal of Cancer*, 45 (1990): 69–76.

Freudenheim, J., et al. "A case-control study of diet and rectal cancer in western New York," in *American Journal of Epidemiology*, 131 (1990): 612–24.

Goldbohm, R. A., et al. "Meat consumption and the risk of colon cancer," in *Cancer Research*, 54(3) (1994): 718–23.

Willett, W. C. "Diet and health: What should we eat?" in *Science*, 264 (1994): 532–37.

Willett, W. C., et al. "Relation of meat, fat, and fiber intake to the risk of colon cancer in a prospective study among women," in *New England Journal of Medicine*, 323 (1990): 1664–72.

On Skin Cancer

Black, H. S. "Effect of a low-fat diet on the incidence of actinic keratosis," in *New England Journal of Medecine*, 330 (1994): 1272–75.

On Prostate Cancer

Francheschi, S. "Fat and prostate cancer," in *Epidemiology*, 5(3) (1994): 271–73.

Le Marchand, L., et al. "Animal fat consumption and prostate cancer: a prospective study in Hawaii," in *Epidemiology*, 5 (1994): 276–82.

Slattery, M. L., et al. "Food – consumption trends between adolescent and adult years and subsequent risk for prostate cancer," in *American Journal of Clinical Nutrition*, 52 (1990): 752–57.

On Pancreatic Cancer

Lyon, J. L., et al. "Dietary intake as a risk factor for cancer of the exocrine pancreas," in *Cancer Epidemiology, Biomakers & Prevention*, 2(6) (1993): 513–18.

On Excessive Amount of Vegetable Fats and Cancer

Carroll, K. K., and H. T. Khor. "Dietary fat in relation to tumorigenesis," in *Progress in Biochemical Pharmacology*, 10 (1975): 308–53.

——— "Effects of level and type of dietary fat on incidence of mammary tumors induced in female Sprague-Dawley rats by 7,12-dimethylbenz (a) antracene," in *Lipids*, 6(6) (1971): 415–20.

On Other Diseases of the Immune System

Chandra, R. K. "1990 McCollum Award Lecture. Nutrition and immunity: lessons from the past and new insights into the future," in *American Journal of Clinical Nutrition*, 53 (1991): 1087–1101.

Cunnane, S. C., et al. "Essential fatty acid and lipid profiles in plasma and erythrocytes in patients with multiple sclerosis," in *American Journal of Clinical Nutrition*, 50 (1989): 801–6.

Darsham, S. K., et al. "Dietary, alpha-linolenic acid and immunocompetence in humans," in *American Journal of Clinical Nutrition*, 53 (1991): 40–46.

Enig, M. G. "Trans-fatty acids — an update," in *Nutrition Quarterly*, 17(4) (1993): 79–95

Kjeldsen-Kragh, J., et al. "Controlled trial of fasting and one-year vegetarian diet in rheumatoid arthritis," in *Lancet*, 338 (1991): 899–902.

Recht, L., et al. "Hand handicap and rheumatoid arthritis in a fish-eating society (the Faroe Islands)," in *Journal of International Medicine*, 227 (1990): 49–55.

Kojima, T., et al. "Long-term administration of highly purified eicosapentaenoic acid provides improvement of psoriasis," in *Dermatologica*, 182 (1991): 225–30.

Walton, A. J., et al. "Dietary fish oil and the severity of symptoms in patients with systemic lupus erythematosus," in *Annals of Rheumatic Diseases*, 50 (1991): 463–66.

On Statistics for Weight Problems

PiSunyer, F. X. "The fattening of America," in *Journal of the American Medical Association*, 272(3) (1994): 238.

On Excess Weight and Health Consequences

Stallone, D. D. "The influence of obesity and its treatment on the immune system," in *Nutrition Reviews*, 52(2, part1) (1994): 37–50.

On Higher Fat Intake Plays a Role

Boozer, C. N., et al. "Dietary fat affects weight loss and adiposity during energy restriction in rats," in *American Journal of Clinical Nutrition*, 58 (1993): 846–52.

Dulloo, A., and L. Girardier. "Adaptive changes in energy expenditure during refeeding following low-calorie intake: evidence for a specific metabolic component favoring fat storage," in *American Journal of Clinical Nutrition*, 52 (1990): 415–20.

Dreon, D., et al. "Dietary fat: carbohydrate ratio and obesity in middle-aged men," in *American Journal of Clinical Nutrition*, 47 (1988): 995–1000.

Hill, J., et al. "Nutrient balances in humans: effects of diet composition," in *American Journal of Clinical Nutrition*, 54 (1992): 10–17.

McKinney, S., and M. S. Buccacio. "Influence of dietary intake on body mass index and body fat of physically active middle-aged males," in *Journal of American Dietetic Association*, 91 (suppl.) (1991): A–100.

Miller, W. C., et al. "Diet composition, energy intake, and exercise in relation to body fat in men and women," in *American Journal of Clinical Nutrition*, 52 (1990): 426–30.

Prewitt E. L., et al. "Changes in body weight, body composition and energy intake in women fed high and low fat diets," in *American Journal of Clinical Nutrition*, 54 (1991): 304–310.

Schutz, Y., et al. "Failure of dietary fat intake to promote fat oxidation; a factor favoring the development of obesity," in *American Journal of Clinical Nutrition*, 50 (1989): 307–14.

Sheppard L., et al. "Weight loss in women participating in a randomized trial of low fat diets," in *American Journal of Clinical Nutrition*, 54 (1991): 821–828.

Stunkard, A. J., et al. "The body-mass index of twins who have been reared apart," in *New England Journal of Medicine*, 322 (1990): 1483–87.

Swinburn B., and E. Ravussin. "Energy balance or fat balance?" in *American Journal of Clinical Nutrition*, 57 (suppl.) (1993): 766–771.

Tremblay, A., et al. "Impact of dietary fat content and fat oxidation on energy intake in humans," in *American Journal of Clinical Nutrition*, 49 (1989): 799–805.

——— "Nutritional determinants of the increase in energy intake associated with a high-fat diet," in *American Journal of Clinical Nutrition*, 53 (1991): 1134–37.

Westerterp, K. R. "Food quotient, respiratory quotient and energy balance," in *American Journal of Clinical Nutrition*, 57 (suppl.) (1993): 759–765.

On Quality of Fat Also Plays a Role

Mann, G. "Metabolic consequences of dietary trans fatty acids," in *Lancet*, 343 (1994): 1268–71.

Pan, D. A., and L. H. Storlien. "Dietary lipid profile is a determinant of tissue phospholipid fatty acid composition and rate of weight gain in rats," in *Journal of Nutrition*, 123 (1993): 512–19.

CHAPTER 3

On Blood Cholesterol and Lipid Profiles

The Canadian Dietetic Association. "Towards healthy blood cholesterol levels — a dietary approach," in *Journal of the Canadian Dietetic Association*, 49 (1988): 216–28.

Cohen, J., et al. "Serum triglycerides' response to fatty meals," in *American Journal of Clinical Nutrition*, 47 (1988): 825–27.

Cominachi, L., et al. "Long-term effect of a low-fat, high-carbohydrate diet on plasma lipids of patients affected by familial endogenous hypertriglyceridemy," in *American Journal of Clinical Nutrition*, 48 (1988): 57–65.

Edington, J., et al. "Serum lipid response to dietary cholesterol in subjects fed a low-fat, high-fiber diet," in *American Journal of Clinical Nutrition*, 50 (1989): 58–62.

Ernst, N. D., and J. Cleeman. "Reducing high blood cholesterol levels: Recommendations from the National Cholesterol Education Program," in *Journal of Nutrition Education*, 20 (1988): 23–29.

Heart and Stroke Foundation of Quebec and Société québecoise de biochimie clinique. *Cholesterol: Results that Are Accurate, Results You Can Trust*, Merck Frosst Canada Inc., 1992.

Kant, K. A., and A. Schatzkin. "Consumption of energy-dense, nutrient-poor foods by the U.S. population: effect on nutient profiles," in *Journal of the American College of Nutrition*, 13(3) (1994): 285–91.

Kasim, S. E., et al. "Dietary and anthropometric determinants of plasma lipoproteins during a long-term low-fat diet in healthy men," in *American Journal of Clinical Nutrition*, 57 (1993): 146–53.

Miettinen, T. A., and Y. A. Kisänumi. "Cholesterol absorption: regulation of cholesterol synthesis and elimination within-populations variations of serum cholesterol levels," in *American Journal of Clinical Nutrition*, 49 (1989): 629–35.

On Low HDL and Normal Total Cholesterol Levels: Not Necessarily a Risk of Heart Disease

Luepker, R. V., et al. "Isolated low HDL-cholesterol as a risk factor for coronary heart disease," in *Circulation*, 88 (suppl.) (1993): 11–511.

On Unblocking the Arteries Is Even More Important

Ornish, D., et al. "Adherence to lifestyle changes and reversal of coronary atherosclerosis," in *Circulation*, 80(4) (1989): 11–57.

———— "Can lifestyle changes reverse coronary heart disease?" in *Lancet*, 336 (1990): 129–33.

CHAPTER 4

On Saturated Fats

Barr, S. L., et al. "Reducing total dietary fat without reducing saturated fatty acids does not significantly lower total plasma cholesterol concentrations in normal males," in *American Journal of Clinical Nutrition*, 55 (1992): 675–81.

Grundy, S. M., and G. V. Vega. "Plasma cholesterol responsiveness to saturated fatty acids," in *American Journal of Clinical Nutrition*, 47 (1988): 822–24.

Hayes, K. C., et al. "Dietary saturated fatty acids (12:0, 14:0, 16:0) differ in their impact on plasma cholesterol and lipoproteins in nonhuman primates," in *American Journal of Clinical Nutrition*, 53 (1991): 491–98.

On Monounsaturated Fats

Baggio, B., et al. "Olive-oil enriched diet: effect on serum lipoprotein levels and biliary cholesterol saturation," in *American Journal of Clinical Nutrition*, 47 (1988) 960–64.

Barradas, M. A., et al. "The effect of olive oil supplementation on human platelet function, serum cholesterol-related variables and plasma fibrinogen concentrations; a pilot study," in *Nutrition Research*, 10 (1990): 403–11.

Grundy, S. M., et al. "Comparison of monounsaturated fatty acids and carbohydrates for reducing raised levels of plasma cholesterol in man," in *American Journal of Clinical Nutrition*, 47 (1988): 965–69.

Parillo, M., et al. "A high monounsaturated-fat/low-carbohydrate diet improves peripheral insulin sensitivity in non-insulin-dependant diabetic patients," in *Metabolism*, 41 (1992): 1371–78.

On Polyunsaturated Fats

Chan, J. K., et al. "Dietary alphalinolenic acid is as effective as oleic acid and linoleic acid in lowering blood cholesterol in normolipidemic men," in *American Journal of Clinical Nutrition*, 53 (1991): 1230–34.

Fumeron, F., et al. "Lowering of HDL2 Cholesterol and lipoprotein A-1 particle levels by increasing the ratio of polyunsaturated to saturated fatty acids," in *American Journal of Clinical Nutrition*, 53 (1991) 655–59.

———— "N-3 polyunsaturated fatty acids raise low-density lipoproteins, high-density lipoprotein 2, and plasminogen activator inhibitor in healthy young men," in *American Journal of Clinical Nutrition*, 54 (1991): 118–22.

Rassias, G., et al. "Linoleic acid lowers LDL cholesterol without a proportionate displacement of saturated fatty acids," in *European Journal of Clinical Nutrition*, 45 (1991): 315–20.

On Omega-3 Fatty Acids

Blonk, M. C., et al. "Dose-response effect of fish-oil supplementation in healthy volunteers," in *American Journal of Clinical Nutrition*, 52 (1990): 120–27.

Bonaa, K. H., et al. "Effect of eicosapentaenoic and docosahexeanoic acids on blood pressure in hypertension. A population-based intervention trial from the Tromsø Study," in *New England Journal of Medicine*, 322 (1990): 795–801.

Brown, A. J., et al. "A mixed Austrialian fish diet and fish-oil supplementation: impact on the plasma lipid profile of healthy men," in *American Journal of Clinical Nutrition*, 52 (1990): 825–33.

Childs, M. T., et al. "Effects of shellfish consumption on lipoproteins in normolipidemic men," in *American Journal of Clinical Nutrition*, 51 (1990): 1020–27.

———— "Divergent lipoprotein response to fish oils with various ratios of eicosapentaenoic acid and docosahexaenoic acid," in *American Journal of Clinical Nutrition*, 52 (1990): 632–39.

Cobiac, L., et al. "Lipid, lipoprotein, and hemostatic effects of fish vs fish oil n-3 fatty acids in mildly hyperlipidemic males," in *American Journal of Clinical Nutrition*, 53 (1991): 1210–16.

Flaten, H., et al. "Fish-oil concentrate: Effects on variables related to cardiovascular disease," in *American Journal of Clinical Nutrition*, 52 (1990): 300–306.

Green, P., et al. "Effects of fish-oil ingestion on cardiovascular risk factors in hyperlipidemic subjects in Israel: a randomized, double-blind crossover study," in *American Journal of Clinical Nutrition*, 52 (1990): 1118–24.

Harris, W. S., et al. "Fish oils in hypertriglyceridemia: a dose-response study," in *American Journal of Clinical Nutrition*, 51 (1990): 399–406.

Kestin, M., et al. "N-3 fatty acids of marine origin lower systolic blood pressure and triglycerides but raise LDL cholesterol compared with n-3 and n-6 fatty acids from plants," in *American Journal of Clinical Nutrition*, 51 (1990): 1028–34.

Margolin, G., et al. "Blood pressure lowering in elderly subjects; a double-blind crossover study of omega-3 and omega-6 fatty acid," in *American Journal of Clinical Nutrition*, 53 (1991): 562–72.

Mori, T. A., et al. "Effect of varying dietary fat, fish, and fish oils on blood lipids in a randomized controlled trial in men at risk of heart disease," in *American Journal of Clinical Nutrition*, 59 (1994): 1060–68.

Silverman, D. I., et al. "Comparison of the absorption and effect on platelet function of a single dose of n-3 fatty acids given as fish or fish oil," in *American Journal of Clinical Nutrition*, 53 (1991): 1165–70.

Van Houvelingen, R., et al. "Dietary fish effects on serum lipids and apolipoproteins, a controlled study," in *American Journal of Clinical Nutrition*, 51 (1990): 393–98.

On *Trans*-fatty Acids

Chardigny, J. M., et al. "Possible physiological effects of *trans*-polyunsaturated fatty acids," in *Essential Fatty Acids and Eicosanoids*. Champaign, Ill: American Oil Chemists' Society, 1992: 148–52.

Enig, M.G. "*Trans*-fatty acids — an update," in *Nutrition Quarterly*, 17(4) (1993): 79–95.

Grundy, S. M. "*Trans*-monounsaturated fatty acids and serum cholesterol levels," in *New England Journal of Medicine*, 323 (1990): 480–81.

Holub, B. J. "Cholesterol-free foods: Where's the *trans?*" in *Canadian Medical Association Journal*, 144 (1991): 3.

Hudgins, L. C., et al. "Correlation of isomeric fatty acids in human adipose tissue with clinical risk factors for cardiovascular disease," in *American Journal of Clinical Nutrition*, 53 (1991): 474–82.

Judd, J. T. "Dietary *trans*-fatty acids: effects on plasma lipids and lipoproteins of healthy men and women," in *American Journal of Clinical Nutrition*, 59 (1994): 861–68.

Koletzko, B. "*Trans*-fatty acids may impair biosynthesis of long-chain polyunsaturates and growth in man," in *Acta Paediatrica*, 81 (1992): 302–306.

Nestel, P., et al. "Plasma lipoprotein lipid and Lp(a) changes with substitution of elaidic for oleic acid in the diet," in *Journal of Lipid Research*, 33 (1992): 1029–36.

Mann, G. "Metabolic consequences of dietary *trans*-fatty acids," in *Lancet*, 343 (1994): 1268–71.

Mensink, R. P., and M. B. Katan. "Effect of dietary *trans*-fatty acids on high-density and low-density lipoprotein cholesterol levels in healthy subjects," in *New England Journal of Medicine*, 323 (1990): 439–45.

Ratnayake, W. M. N., and G. Pelletier. "Positional and geometrical isomers of linoleic acid in partially hdrogenated oils," in *Journal of the American Oil Chemists' Society*, 69(2) (1992): 95–105.

Ratnayake, W. M. N., et al. "Fatty acids in some common foods items in Canada," in *Journal of the American College of Nutrition*, 12(6) (1993): 651–60.

Troisi, R., et al. "*Trans*-fatty acid intake in relation to serum lipid concentrations in adult men," in *American Journal of Clinical Nutrition*, 56 (1992): 1019–24.

Willett, W. C., et al. "Intake of *trans*-fatty acids and risk of coronary heart disease among women," in *Lancet*, 341 (1993): 581–85.

Willet, W. C., and A. Ascherio. "*Trans*-fatty acids: Are the effects only marginal?" in *American Journal of Public Health*, 84(5) (1994): 1–3.

Wood, R., et al. "Effect of butter, mono- and polyunsaturated fatty acid-enriched butter, *trans*-fatty acid margarine, and zero *trans*-fatty acid margarine on serum lipids and lipoproteins in healthy men," in *Journal of Lipid Research*, 34 (1993): 1–11.

Zock, P. L., and M. B. Katan. "Hydrogenation alternatives: effects of *trans*-fatty acids and stearic acid versus linleic acid on serum lipids and lipoproteins in humans," in *Journal of Lipid Research*, 33 (1992): 399–410.

On the Nutritional Value of Foods

Brault Dubuc, M., and L. Caron Lahaie. *Nutritive value of foods.* Québec: Brault-Lahaie Edition, 1994.

Health and Welfare Canada. *Nutrient Value of Some Common Foods.* Ottawa: Minister of Supply and Services Canada, 1987.

Human Nutrition Information Service. *Composition of Foods. Handbook No. 8 series.* Washington: United States Department of Agriculture, 1976–86.

Simopoulos, A. P., et al. "Common purslane: A source of omega-3 fatty acids and antioxidants," in *Journal of the American College of Nutrition*, 11(4) (1992): 374–82.

CHAPTER 5

On Eating Trends over the Years

Eaton, S. B., and M. Konner. "Paleolithic nutrition," in *New England Journal of Medicine*, 312 (5) (1985): 283–89.

Beggs, L., et al. "Tracking nutrition trends: Canadians' attitudes, knowledge and behaviours regarding fat, fibre and cholesterol," in *Journal of Canadian Dietetic Association*, 54 (1993): 21–28.

Gagnon, G., and B. Shateinstein. *Consommation lipidique des résidents du Montréal métropolitain.* Montreal: Département de santé communautaire, Hôpital général de Montréal, 1989.

Santé Québec. *Enquête québécoise sur la nutrition, 1990. Résultats préliminaires de l'enquête.* Quebec: Santé Québec, 1994.

Slattery, M. L., and D. E. Randall. "Trends in coronary heart disease mortality and food consumption in the United States between 1909 and 1980," in *American Journal of Clinical Nutrition*, 47 (1988): 1060–67.

Stephen, A. M., and N. J. Wald. "Trends in individual consumption of dietary fat in the United States 1920–1984," in *American Journal of Clinical Nutrition*, 52 (1990): 457–69.

On Current Recommendations and Their Limits

Health and Welfare Canada. *Nutrition Recommendations: The Report of the Scientific Review Committee.* Ottawa: Minister of Supply and Services Canada, 1990.

McDonald, B. *Dietary Fat: Fine-tuning the Message.* Ottawa: National Institute of Nutrition, Review no. 20, 1993.

On the Type of Fat Has More Impact on Health Than the 30 Percent Limit

Colquhoun, D. M. "Comparison of the effects on lipoproteins and apolipoproteins of a diet high in monounsaturated fatty acids enriched with avocado and a high carbohydrate diet," in *American Journal of Clinical Nutrition,* 56 (1992): 671–77.

Hasegawa, K., et al. "Nutritional assessment trial (fatty acids in particular) in community health and nutrition in Japan," in *The Third International Congress on Essential Fatty Acids and Eicosanoids,* American Oil Chemists' Society, (1992): 81–83.

Junshi, C., C. T. Campbell, et al. *Diet, Life-style and Mortality in China.* Oxford: Oxford University Press, 1990.

Mata, P., et al. "Effect of dietary monounsaturated fatty acids on plasma lipoproteins and apolipoproteins in women," in *American Journal of Clinical Nutrition,* 56 (1992): 77–83.

Ornish, D., et al. "Adherence to lifestyle changes and reversal of coronary atherosclerosis," in *Circulation,* 80(4) (1989): 11–57.

––––––– "Can lifestyle changes reverse coronary heart disease?" in *Lancet,* 336 (1990): 129–33.

Spiller G. A., et al. "Effect of a diet high in monounsaturated fat from almonds on plasma cholesterol and lipoproteins," in *Journal of the American College of Nutrition,* 11 (1992): 126–30.

Wardlaw, M. G., and J. T. Snook. "Effect of diet high in butter, corn oil, or high oleic-acid sunflower oil on serum lipids and lipoproteins in men," in *American Journal of Clinical Nutrition,* 51 (1990): 815–21.

Wardlaw, M. G., and al. "Serum lipid and lipoprotein concentrations in healthy men on diets enriched in either canola oil or safflower oil," in *American Journal of Clinical Nutrition*, 54 (1991): 104–10.

On the French Paradox

Frankel, E. N., et al. "Inhibition of oxidation of human low-density lipoprotein by phenolic substances in red wine," in *Lancet*, 341 (1993): 454–47.

Gander, K. F. "Fats in the diet," in *Journal of American Oil Chemists' Society*, 53 (1976): 417.

Mann, G. "Metabolic consequences of dietary trans fatty acids," in *Lancet*, 343 (1994): 1268–71.

Renaud, S. C., et al. "Wine, alcohol, platelets and the French paradox for coronary heart disease," in *Lancet*, 339 (1992): 1523–26.

———— "Alcohol and platelet aggregation: the caerphilly prospective heart disease study," in *American Journal of Clinical Nutrition*, 55 (1992): 1012–17.

On Our Basic Needs

Health and Welfare Canada. *Nutrition Recommendations: The Report of the Scientific Review Committee.* Ottawa: Minister of Supply and Services Canada, 1990.

Gronn, M., et al. "Dietary n-6 fatty acids inhibit the incorporation of dietary n-3 fatty acids in thrombocyte and serum phospholipids in humans: a controlled dietetic study," in *Scandinavia Journal of Clinical Laboratory Investigation*, 51 (1991): 255–63.

On the Good Fats

Hunter, J. E. "N-3 fatty acids from vegetable oils," in *American Journal of Clinical Nutrition*, 51 (1990): 809–14.

Jacotot, B. *L'huile d'olive de la gastronomie à la santé.* Paris: Éditions Artulen, 1993.

Mata, P., et al. "Effect of dietary monounsaturated fatty acids on plasma lipoproteins and apolipoproteins in women," in *American Journal of Clinical Nutrition*, 56 (1992): 77–83.

Polyunsaturated Fats and Oxidation

Kubow S. "Routes of formation and toxic consequences of lipid oxidation products in foods," in *Free Radical Biology and Medicine*, 12 (1992): 63–81.

On Tropical Oils

Cottrel, R. C. "Introduction: nutritional aspects of palm oil," in *American Journal of Clinical Nutrition*, 53 (1991): S989–1009.

Chakrabarty, M. M. "Carotene from red palm oil: current status, future possibilities in combating vitamin A deficiency through dietary improvement," in *Nutrition Foundation of India*, Special publication series 6, 1992.

Tholstrup, T., et al. "Fat high in stearic acid favorably affects blood lipids and factor VII coagulant activity in comparison with fats high in palmitic acid of high in myristic and lauric acids," in *American Journal of Clinical Nutrition*, 59 (1994): 371–77.

On Fat Intake in Europe in 1975

Formo W. M., et al. *Bailey's Industrial Oil and Fat Products,* 4th Edition. Toronto: Daniel Swern, vol. 1, 1979 and vol. 2, 1982.

On Nutritional Content of Foods

Brault Dubuc, M., and L. Caron Lahaie. *Nutritive Value of Foods.* Quebec: Brault-Lahaie Edition, 1994.

Human Nutrition Information Service. *Composition of Foods — Handbook no. 8 series*. Washington: United States Department of Agriculture, 1976–86.

McCance and Widdowson's. *The Composition of Foods. First Supplement on Amino Acid Composition and Fatty Acid Composition*. London: Royal Society of Chemistry, 1980.

Health and Welfare Canada. *Nutrient Value of Some Common Foods*. Ottawa: Ministry of Supply and Services, 1987.

CHAPTER 6

On Canadian Labeling

Consumer and Corporate Affairs Canada. *Guide for Food Manufacturers and Advertisers*. Ottawa: Consumer Products Branch, 1988.

Health and Welfare Canada. *Guidelines for Health Information Programs Involving the Sales of Foods*. Ottawa: Food Directorate, Health Protection Branch, 1991.

National Institute of Nutrition. *Consumer Use and Understanding of Nutrition Information on Food Labels*. Ottawa: National Institute of Nutrition, 1992.

On Nutritional Content of Foods

Canadian Diabetic Association. *Food choices in the market place*. 1987.

Brault Dubuc, M., and L. Caron Lahaie. *Nutritive Value of Foods*. Quebec: Brault-Lahaie Edition, 1994.

Kraft General Foods. *L'analyse nutritionnelle des produits d'épicerie*. Kraft General Foods.

CHAPTER 7

On Margarines

Booyens J., et al. "Margarines and coronary heart disease," in *Medical Hypotheses*, 37 (1992): 241–44.

Ratnayake, R., et al. "Fatty acids in Canadian margarines," in *Canadian Institute of Food Science and Technology*, 24 (1–2) (1991): 81–86.

Wolff, R. L. "Trans-polyunsaturated fatty acids in French edible rapeseed and soybean oils," in *Journal of the American Oil Chemists' Society*, 69 (2) (1992): 106–10.

On Cold-pressed Oils

Becker, M., et al. "Long-term treatment of severe familial hypercholesterolemia in children: Effect of sitosterol and bezafibrate," in *Pediatrics*, 89 (1992): 138–142.

Beveridge, J. M. R., et al. "Magnitude of the hypocholesterolemic effect of dietary sitosterol in man," in *Journal of Nutrition*, 83 (1964): 119–22.

Bracco, U., et al. "Production and use of natural antioxidants," in *Journal of the American Oil Chemists' Society*, 58(6) (1981): 686–90.

Chandler, et al. "Antihypercholesterolemic studies with sterols: ß-sitosterol and stigmasterol," in *Journal of Pharmaceutical Sciences*, 68(2) (1979): 245–47.

Drieu, F. "Études comparatives sur les huiles de tournesol, compte-rendu des analyses effectuées au Laboratoire de la Direction Générale de la Concurrence, de la Consommation et de la Répression des fraudes à Montpellier," *Bulletin de l'AMKI*, 1 (1991): 16–19.

Heinemann, G. A., et al. "Mechanisms of action of plant sterols on inhibition of cholesterol absorption," in *European Journal of Pharmacology*, 40 (suppl.) (1991): S59–S63.

Lambert-Lagacé, L., and D. Lamontagne. "Les huiles pressées à froid," in *Diététique en action*, 4(1) (1990): 23–25.

Lees, A. M., et al. "Plant sterols as cholesterol-lowering agents: clinical trials in patients with hypercholesterolemia and studies of sterol balance," in *Artherosclerosis*, 28 (1977): 325–38.

Packer, L. "Protective role of vitamin E in biological systems," in *American Journal of Clinical Nutrition*, 53 (1991): 1050S–55S.

Salen, G., et al. "Metabolism of ß-Sitosterol in Man," in *The Journal of Clinical Investigation*, 49 (1970): 952–67.

On Canola Oil

Gustafsson, I. B., et al. "A diet rich in monounsaturated rapeseed oil reduces the lipoprotein cholesterol concentration and increases the relative content of n-3 fatty acids in serum in hyperlipidemic subjects," in *American Journal of Clinical Nutrition*, 59 (1994): 667–74.

On Olive Oil

De Bruin, T. W. A., et al. "Different postprandial metabolism of olive oil and soybean oil: A possible mechanism of the high density lipoprotein conserving effect of olive oil," in *American Journal of Clinical Nutrition*, 58 (1993): 477–83.

Fedeli, E. "Lipids of olives," in *Progress in Chemistry*, 15 (1977): 57–74.

On Walnut Oil

Abbey, M., et al. "Partial replacement of saturated fatty acids with almonds and walnuts lowers total plasma cholesterol and low-density-lipoprotein cholesterol," in *American Journal of Clinical Nutrition*, 59 (1994): 995–99.

On Tropical Oils

Cottrel, R. C. "Introduction: Nutritional aspects of palm oil," in *American Journal of Clinical Nutrition*, 53 (1991): S989–1009.

Chakrabarty, M. M. "Carotene from red palm oil: current status, future possibilities in combating vitamin A deficiency through dietary improvement," in *Nutrition Foundation of India*, Special publication series 6, 1992.

Tholstrup, T., et al. "Fat high in stearic acid favorably affects blood lipids and factor VII coagulant activity in comparison with fats high in palmitic acid of high in myristic and lauric acids," in *American Journal of Clinical Nutrition*, 59 (1994): 371–77.

CHAPTER 8

On the Impact of Gamma-linolenic Acid

Gunstone, F. D. "Gamma-linolenic acid occurrence and physical and chemical properties," in *Progress in Lipid Research*, 31 (1992): 141–56.

Horrobin, D. F. "Nutritional and medical importance of gamma-linolenic acid," in *Progress in Lipid Research*, 31 (1992): 163–94.

———— "Fatty acid metabolism in health and disease: the role of delta 6 desaturase," in *American Journal of Clinical Nutrition*, 57 (suppl.) (1993): 732S–37S.

Evening Primrose Oil Supplements

Drieu-Gervois, F. "Contrôle des huiles d'onagre, compte-rendu des analyses effectuées au Laboratoire de la Direction Générale de la Concurrence, de la Consommation et de la Répression des fraudes à Montpellier," *Bulletin de l'AMKI*, 3 (1992,): 9–21.

On Fish Oils

Burr, M. L., et al. "Effects of changes in fat, fish, and fibre intakes on death and myocardial reinfarction: diet and reinfarction trial (DART)," in *Lancet*, (1989): 757–61.

Haglund, O., et al. "Effects of a new fluid fish oil concentrate, Eskimo-3, on triglycerides, cholesterol, fibrinogen and blood pressure," in *Journal of Internal Medicine*, 227 (1990): 347–53.

Kinsella, J. E. *Seafoods and Fish Oils in Human Health and Disease*. New York: Marcel Dekker, Inc., 1987.

Stenson W. F., et al. "Dietary supplementation with fish oil in ulcerative colitis," in *Annals of Internal Medicine*, 116 (1992): 609–14.

Vilaseca, J., et al. "Dietary fish oil reduces progression of chronic inflammatory lesions in rat model of granulomatous colitis," in *Gut*, 31 (1990): 539–44.

On Fat Substitutes

Smith, R. E., et al. "Overview of Salatrim, a family of low-calorie fats," in *Journal of Agricultural and Food Chemistry*, 42 (2) (1994): 432–41.

Vanderveen, J. E., and W. H. Glinsmann. "Fat substitutes: a regulatory perspective," in *Annual Review of Nutrition*, 12 (1992): 473–487.

CHAPTER 9

On Culinary Tips

The Magazine of Food & Health: Eating Well, 1992–94.

Canadian Living, 1990–94.

INDEX